N. I. Raspopowa
M. Ju. Lübchenko

DIAGNOSIS AND THERAPY OF ANXIETY-DEPRESSIVE DISORDERS

N. I. Raspopowa
M. Ju. Lübchenko

DIAGNOSIS AND THERAPY OF ANXIETY-DEPRESSIVE DISORDERS

WITH SLEEP DISORDERS IN PRIMARY CARE SETTINGS

ScienciaScripts

Imprint
Any brand names and product names mentioned in this book are subject to trademark, brand or patent protection and are trademarks or registered trademarks of their respective holders. The use of brand names, product names, common names, trade names, product descriptions etc. even without a particular marking in this work is in no way to be construed to mean that such names may be regarded as unrestricted in respect of trademark and brand protection legislation and could thus be used by anyone.

Cover image: www.ingimage.com

This book is a translation from the original published under ISBN 978-620-3-20040-9.

Publisher:
Sciencia Scripts
is a trademark of
International Book Market Service Ltd., member of OmniScriptum Publishing Group
17 Meldrum Street, Beau Bassin 71504, Mauritius
Printed at: see last page
ISBN: 978-620-3-18436-5

MINISTRY OF HEALTH AND SOCIAL DEVELOPMENT OF THE
REPUBLIC OF KAZAKHSTAN

KAZAKH MEDICAL UNIVERSITY OF CONTINUING EDUCATION
KARAGANDA STATE MEDICAL UNIVERSITY

Raspopova N.I., Lyubchenko M.Y.

DIAGNOSIS AND THERAPY OF ANXIETY-DEPRESSIVE DISORDERS WITH SLEEP DISORDERS IN PRIMARY HEALTH CARE

(Textbook)

Almaty, 2020

UDC
616.89
LBC
©

Raspopova N.I., Lyubchenko M.Y. Diagnosis and therapy of anxiety-depressive disorders with sleep disorders in primary care. Training manual - Almaty, 2020, 73 p.
ISBN

Authors: N.I. Raspopova -Professor of the Department of Psychiatry   , Psychotherapy and Narcology, KazMUNO, M.D.

Lubchenko M.Y. - Professor , Department of Neurology, Neurosurgery, Psychiatry and Rehabilitation, Medical University of Karaganda, M.D.

Reviewers:

1. K.S. Altynbekov - Deputy Director for Scientific and Clinical Work, RSPC PZ MH RK, M.D.

2. Abetova A.A. - Head of the Department of Psychiatry, Psychotherapy and Narcology, KazMUNO, Candidate of Medical Sciences.

The problems of diagnosis and therapy of depressive conditions occupy one of the leading places in clinical psychiatry. In spite of the fact that depression is a mental disorder, the majority of depressive disorders are not in the field of vision of a psychiatrist, and these patients are observed by general practitioners. The textbook presents contemporary theoretical aspects of the etiopathogenesis of anxiety-depressive disorders and their classification. The features of diagnostics of depression, variants of its comorbidity with somatic pathology among patients of the general medical practice are singled out. Modern approaches to the therapy of sleep disorders in depressions detected in patients attending primary health care institutions are described.

The textbook is intended for use in the curricula of medical schools and postgraduate medical education, as well as for practicing physicians psychiatrists, psychotherapists, neurologists, medical psychologists and general practitioners.

© Raspopova N.I., Lyubchenko M.Y.
2020

Contents

Introduction

A sad, depressed mood can normally be considered a normal human emotional reaction to stressful events, disappointment or loss in life. However, depressed moods, sadness can manifest itself in the structure of a severe mental illness of the affective sphere - depression. Recent epidemiological studies show that one in eight people at least once in their lifetime requires special antidepressant or thymoanaleptic therapy for depression. Depression causes the strongest psychological, emotional and physical suffering, which significantly reduces the quality of life of the patient, the level of his family, social and labor adaptation, and often leads to disability. Depression often goes hand in hand with somatic diseases and always complicates their prognosis. But the most terrible consequence of depression is suicide, which is committed by about 15% of patients [1].

The terminological definition of depression has a rather wide range of states, represented both by a temporary decrease in mood of a situational nature, and by a psychopathological symptom accompanied by hypothymia, combined with ideational and motor retardation, specific vital feelings, insomnia, decreased concentration , anhedronia, vegetative disorders, pessimistic orientation of thinking. Depression can also be presented as a mental illness, manifesting as a recurrence of the syndrome in an expanded or reduced form with a decrease in the level of social adaptation. Recent data on the prevalence of mental disorders in Europe show that they are newly detected in 83 million people each year, with depressive disorders accounting for 68% of mental illnesses. Some researchers have noted that while the prevalence of mental disorders has been relatively stable, there has been a steady increase in the incidence of depression (2,3).

The reasons for such a significant increase in the prevalence of depressive disorders are primarily rooted in changes in people's social structures and living conditions: the destruction of the institution of marriage, the weakening of family ties, the unrelenting pace of scientific and technological progress. Causal factors also include an orientation toward material consumption to the detriment of spiritual interests, loneliness and social isolation, in which the elderly in particular often find themselves today. Finally, an increase in life expectancy in almost all countries of the world plays a role, because old age, in which somatic diseases (cardiovascular diseases, cancer) are more frequent, is also a risk factor for depressive disorders [4,5]. Many researchers point out in their works, that over the past 100 years no new clinical forms of depression have appeared, but the

The dynamics of the course of depression. The number of prolonged depressions lasting up to two years has increased from 20 to 45% of cases [6]. In 10-18% of cases, in spite of adequate therapy, depressions acquire a chronic course. In 45% of patients, only short-term (up to 6 months) remissions occur [7,8]. At the same time, in 70-85% of patients who have had a depressive

episode, relapses subsequently develop, in the first year of remission in 21% of patients, in the second year - in 32% and in the third year of remission
- in 35% of patients. Repeated, within one year, hospital admissions for depressed patients increased from 6 to 29%. Severe forms of depression affect 5% of the population. The significance of depression is determined by the nature of its course - relapsing or continuous. The marked character of depression is observed in 60% of patients [9,10]. There is evidence that patients who have had 1 depressive episode have a recurrent episode in 50% of cases. In patients who have suffered 3 depressive episodes, there is a risk of suffering a fourth episode in 90% of cases.

Comorbidity of depression with anxiety disorders and somatic pathology is most frequently mentioned as one of the factors of unfavorable clinical and social prognosis of depression in modern studies. According to Y.L. Nuller [11], the chronic course in 71% of depressed patients is associated with comorbid obsessive and hypochondriacal disorders. Depressions combined with panic and phobic disorders also have a protracted course (70% and 77.3% of patients, respectively). At the same time, in 18.3% of the patients, the dynamics of the phobic syndrome has a progredient character [1,12,13].

Despite the fact that depression is a mental disorder, two-thirds of cases do not come to the attention of a psychiatrist and are observed by general practitioners. Cases of severe depression account for 5 to 8% of the total flow of outpatients. Depression can provoke somatic diseases (especially reactive depression), often contributing to the development of hypertension and other pathological changes of internal organs, and be a reaction to them, as well as not depending on the somatic disease, but in all cases, depression aggravates the course of the physical disease and complicates its treatment. Major international studies conducted in 14 medical [13,14].

The adverse effect of depression on the course and prognosis of many somatic diseases, as well as the extensive positive experience of treatment of depression by general practitioners in many countries of the world, are important evidence for the need to eliminate it from the
The "diagnostic invisibles" into the arena of general medical practice. Current scientific evidence and the general trend in the care of patients presenting to various levels of health care for some form of suffering suggest diagnosis and treatment of depressive disorders, starting in the primary care setting (15).

1. Current aspects of the etiology and pathogenesis of depressive disorders

Neurobiological basis of depression. The anatomical bases of emotions are the brain structures belonging to the limbic system: hippocampus with conduction pathways, transparent septum, nuclei of the amygdala complex, cingulate gyrus. Neuromorphological studies have shown enlargement of the lateral ventricles of the brain in depression, which can be interpreted as atrophy of the hippocampus. Disruption of the sleep-wake cycle in depression indicates the involvement in the pathogenesis of a number of nuclei lying in the reticular formation of the trunk, bridge and midbrain. A wide range of autonomic disorders (changes in heart rate, skin and galvanic reactions, electromyogram) observed in depression indicate the involvement of central parts of the autonomic system, hypothalamic-pituitary system in their pathogenesis.

In depressions, there is impairment of a number of cortical functions, such as changes in color perception and emotional facial expressions, impaired eye movement, impaired gaze contact, and slowed motor reactions. Deautomatization of mental functions manifests itself in difficulty thinking, probable forecasting, decision-making. Thus, the morphological substrate of emotions and emotional disorders can be considered practically the whole brain, as well as the neuroendocrine system [13].

Neurochemical basis of depression. A variety of clinical manifestations of depressive disorders, the multiplicity of molecular mechanisms of action of antidepressants of different groups indicate the participation of interrelated disorders of several neurochemical systems in the pathogenesis of depression. Serotonin and norepinephrine deficits in the CNS play a key role in the pathogenesis of depression. In addition, these systems closely interact with the dopaminergic   , cholinergic, melatoninergic, glutamatergic, and GABAergic systems.

Modern studies have proven that monoamine neurotransmitter pathways are relevant to the expression of emotions, the regulation of mood, and the maintenance of the waking state. Serotonin plays an important role in the regulation of emotional behavior, motor activity, eating behavior, sleep, thermoregulation, and is involved in the control of neuroendocrine systems. But despite significant progress in the understanding of the pathogenesis of depression, the chain of its biological mechanisms requires further study. There are data showing that impaired serotonergic transmission does not play a key role in the development of depression, but only reflects one of the stages of the depressive "cascade", in which dysfunction of the hypothalamic-pituitary-adrenal system also has a certain significance.

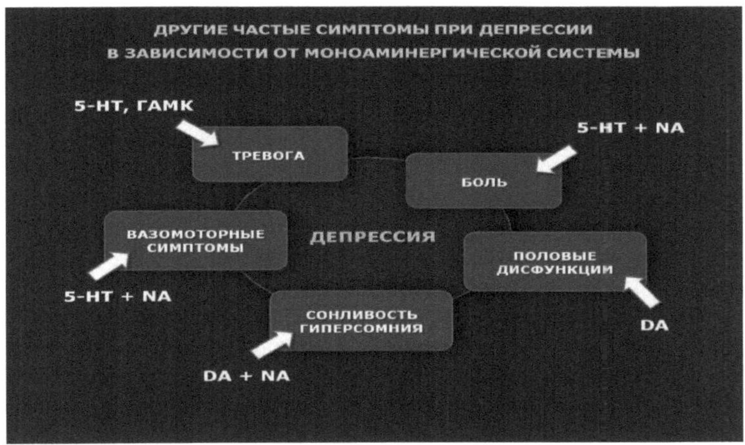

Figure 1 - Symptoms of depression depending on the monoaminergic system

Antidepressants are thought to exert their therapeutic influence by potentiating synaptic transmission at noradrenergic and serotonergic synapses, as well as by influencing the dopamine system. Due to the differences in the efficacy of therapy with different antidepressants, *several neurochemical types of depression are accepted,* related mainly to serotonin deficiency, to serotonin excess but decreased postsynaptic receptor sensitivity, to noradrenaline and serotonin depletion (late-life depression) or to imbalance of these neurotransmitters.

There is a growing body of evidence linking the symptoms of depression with disturbances of biological rhythms, and the symptoms of depression themselves can have a significant impact on the quality of life and well-being of patients. Depression has been found to be characterized by profound disturbances in biological rhythms due to desynchronization of circadian rhythms [17,18]. Symptoms of depression due to circadian rhythm disturbances, such as depressed mood, weakness, loss of energy, urges or interests, and drowsiness, have a significant impact on patients' condition and quality of life, including a decline in professional and social functioning [16,19,20].

Sleep disorders occur with depression and are manifested by difficulty falling asleep, shallow nocturnal sleep, early awakening in the morning. At the same time, in the morning and in the afternoon, patients experience feelings of drowsiness, lethargy and brokenness. Sleep problems are not specific to depressive disorders, but are noted *as one of the most frequent symptoms* of depression. Depressed patients are characterized by a decrease in the total duration of sleep, a significant reduction in its slow stages and a shortening of sleep cycles. The latent period of the first phase of REM sleep is significantly reduced (from 65 minutes in normal to 20 minutes in severe depression), which is one of the biological markers of depression. [21]. In depression, disorders of the circadian rhythm of sleep are represented by a type of delayed and premature sleep phase. The former is characterized by difficulties in initiating and ending sleep at the desired (socially acceptable) time. When the biological sleep-wake rhythm shifts to an earlier time, a circadian sleep rhythm disorder of the type of premature phase of sleep develops. Patients with this disorder are characterized by complaints of early morning and night awakenings with inability to go back to sleep. Ch. Sinton and V. McCarley (2003) found that in classic depressions, a decrease in the latent period of REM sleep is clearly registered [22].

The circadian rhythm governs our internal biological rhythms; it determines the functioning of the entire human body, regulating and directing a variety of biological, physiological, and behavioral processes that manifest themselves in a variety of everyday human functions, including body temperature, blood pressure, mood swings, and the sleep-wake cycle. They are controlled by a biological clock located in the hypothalamus of the human brain [23,24].

Genetic background of depressive disorders. The fact that some emotional disorders manifest themselves as inherited, gives reason to think about the role of genetic factors. The genetic hypothesis of the formation of depressions is largely comparable to the views on the CNS pathology observed by neurologists in diseases accompanied by the processes of apoptosis (Parkinson's disease, Alzheimer's disease and other neurodegenerative diseases). In particular, it is believed that depression is caused by changes in the work of critical genes, the activity of which is stopped due to the deficiency of monoamines - neurotransmitters: serotonin, noradrenaline, dopamine. In this case, the genes stop "issuing commands" for the synthesis of a number of substances necessary for normal neuronal functioning. Accordingly, it is no coincidence that the findings obtained from postmortem brain material of patients with affective disorders indicate that the volume and thickness of the rostral orbitofrontal cortex, prefrontal cortex, anterior cingulate and parahippocampal cortex, as well as the volume of basal ganglia and n.accumbens are reduced compared to the norm [25].

Due to the development of methods of vital structural neuroimaging of the human brain (X-ray computed tomography - CT, magnetic resonance imaging - MRI) it is shown that neuromorphological findings are not artifacts. It is established that in affective disorders the lateral and 3rd ventricles of the brain are enlarged, the volume of gray matter in the frontal, orbitofrontal, medial prefrontal, temporal and parietal cortical areas, ventral striatum and in the hippocampus is reduced. Finally, according to functional neuroimaging data, depressed patients have reduced local cerebral blood flow and glucose metabolism in limbic structures and prefrontal cortex. Genetic factors are of particular importance in endogenous versions of depression. The risk of developing the disease in these cases is estimated to be 10-20% if one parent has the disease, and 4-10% if second-line relatives have the disease [1,26,27].

Psychosocial basis of depressive disorders. There are numerous attempts at a psychosocial interpretation of the mechanism of affective disorders. Freud believed that vulnerability to depression is established in early infancy at the time of feeding, as a result of a traumatic relationship with the mother, characterized by inadequate attention or overly emotional treatment of the child.

An increased dependence on emotionally significant relations with others and constant fear of their loss is formed. The dysphoric reaction to the broken contact with the mother, accompanied by a decrease in self-esteem, is fixed and symbolically reproduced further in similar social situations - most often in actual or assumed loss of an emotionally significant object. Freud believed that the child, feeling aggression toward an emotionally significant person for lack of attention to him or her, can turn that aggression toward him or herself in order not to lose the connection with this person. He considered such a change of aggression direction as a primary or necessary condition for the subsequent development of depression[28].

Loss of parents before the age of 11 has been found to be one of the predicates of the likely occurrence of a depressive episode later on; depressed patients have reliably more psychological trauma (mostly loss of loved ones) in the 6 months preceding the episode than the general population. A depressive state can be caused not only by signals symbolizing loss, but also by direct, direct unmet need, generating a real threat to either health, prestige, or both. Needs are closely connected with emotions, and the richness, complexity and depth, strength and numerous shades of human emotions indicate the variety of needs behind them and characterize individuality. Material - biological, social and ideal needs form complex interconnected complexes that can have a direct impact on the affective sphere [29].

<u>Cognitive theories</u> proceed from the fact that in the course of an illness, as a result of repeated action of social stressors, steady, individual for each patient, so-called depressogenic patterns are formed.

These schemes represent a peculiar circle of automated thought reactions to a stressor and emotional reactions to similar thoughts. The activation of these schemes, which are interconnected with the most important personality traits, can steadily affect self-esteem and social perception, causing a distorted view of the self, the world around and the future ("cognitive triad"). The automatized nature of the affect can lead to a loss of meaningful connection to the stressor in question, the cognitive errors contained in the dysfunctional thoughts cease to be recognized by the patient and the changes of his affective states seem inexplicable. The most typical cognitive errors operating in depressogenic schemes are:

- an arbitrary conclusion drawn without sufficient reason;
- selective fixation on the negative components of the situation while ignoring other elements;
- Exaggeration of the actual significance of negative components with an understatement of positive ones;

- The use of isolated, insignificant episodes to form an inappropriately generalized, distorted view of reality.

Depressed patients tend to see the cause of their failure in themselves rather than in the world around them, to regard the causal factor as stable rather than temporary, acting globally rather than in a limited number of situations (i.e., generalizing, omitting and distorting the internal picture of the world). Failure in everyday life is used by patients as an argument to prove their inability to act successfully in the future, with an accompanying sense of deadlock and futility. This vicious cognitive circle has led to the concept of "learned helplessness." [30,31].

2. Classification and typology of depression

Depression (from Latin depressio - suppression, oppression) is a mental disorder characterized by a pathologically lowered mood (hypothymia) with a negative, pessimistic assessment of oneself, one's position in surrounding reality and one's future. Depressive change of mood, along with distortion of cognitive processes, is accompanied by motor inhibition, a decrease in urges to activity and somatovegetative dysfunctions. Depressive symptomatology negatively affects social adaptation and quality of life. The systematics of depression has traditionally been based on a nosological classification[27,32]. Accordingly, depressions were distinguished within the framework of such mental diseases as manic-depressive psychosis, schizophrenia, psychogenias, etc. The differentiation was carried out within the limits of a classical etiological and clinical dichotomy, defining endogenous or exogenous character of affective disorders.

According to the leading etiological factor, Ponizovsky K.M. [33] distinguishes 3 main nosological categories of depression: ***somatogenic, endogenous, psychogenic.*** Somatogenic refers to depressions caused by somatic (organic) disorders. They are subdivided into *organic*, when the basis of depression is an organic lesion of the brain, and *symptomatic*, in which the depressive state is one of many manifestations of a somatic illness (for example, cancer). Endogenous depression develops mainly on the basis of a hereditary predisposition. These include schizoaffective depression (in schizophrenia), circular or cyclothymic depression (in manic-depressive psychosis), and involutionary depression in the second half of life. Psychogenic depressions are triggered mainly by adverse situational and environmental influences (stress, conflicts). Depressions caused by the loss of a loved one are traditionally called *reactive, and* another kind of psychogenic depression - *neurotic* depression - is caused by an internal contradiction that cannot be solved for the person - the neurotic conflict.

In the modern classification (ICD-10), the main importance is given to variants of the course of depression:

- the only depressing episode
- recurrent depression
- Bipolar disorder (alternating depressive and manic phases)
- cyclothymia
- dysthymia

as well as the severity of depression

- light
- moderate
- Heavy
  Mild depression
  (subdepression) (F.32.0 ICD-

10)

* the main manifestations are weakly expressed

* the clinical picture shows only some monosymptoms - fatigue, unwillingness to do anything, anhedonia, sleep disorders, decreased appetite

* Depressive disorders may be masked by other psychopathological disorders (anxious-phobic, hypochondriacal, vegetative, algic) One symptom dominates in the clinical picture without a pronounced manifestation of the entire affective syndrome

<u>Depression of moderate severity</u> (ICD-10 F.32.1)

* the main manifestations of depression are moderate

* Decreased social and professional functioning

<u>Severe depression</u> (ICD-10 F.32.2)

- severe depression without psychotic manifestations

* either sadness or apathy, psychomotor retardation, anxiety, restlessness dominate, suicidal thoughts and tendencies are revealed

- Severe depression with psychotic manifestations

Delusions of guilt, illness, motor lethargy (up to and including stupor) or agitation [34].

According to a two-level typology of depression, its psychopathological manifestations are subdivided into

- **positive affectivity**
- **negative affectivity**

Positive affectivity is represented in the structure of depressions by the phenomena of the circle of "psychic hyperesthesia" (Korsakov S.S. 1913). Pathological affect is extremely pronounced in vital (wistful) depression, realized as a grievous mental disorder. On the clinical level, the phenomena of affective hyperaesthesia are realized in the form of vital longing. Mopey affect is accompanied by ideas of worthlessness, self-deprecation, and ideational and motor inhibition. Positive affectivity includes the following psychopathological manifestations:

<u>Longing</u> is an indefinite, diffuse (protopathic) feeling in the form of intolerable oppression in the chest or epigastrium, with depression, despondency, hopelessness; it has the character of mental suffering (mental pain, anguish).

<u>Anxiety</u> is unfounded uncertain excitement, a premonition of danger, impending disaster with a feeling of inner tension. It can be perceived as unreasonable anxiety.

<u>Intellectual and motor inhibition</u> - difficulties in concentration, concentration of attention, slowness of reactions, inertness, loss of spontaneous activity.

<u>Pathological circadian rhythm</u> - fluctuations of mood during the day with a maximum of bad feeling in the early morning and some improvement in the afternoon and evening.

<u>Ideas of inferiority, sinfulness, damage</u> - an unremitting reflection on

their own worthlessness, depravity, with a negative revaluation of the past, present, future prospects, the idea of the illusory nature of the real successes achieved, the guilt even in what has not yet been committed.

Suicidal thoughts - psychologically unbearable desire to die with ideas of senselessness of existence, desirability of an accident with a fatal outcome or intention to kill oneself - can take on the character of obsessive ideas, an irresistible attraction to suicide (suicidomania).

Hypochondriacal ideas are dominant ideas about the danger (usually greatly exaggerated) and futility of treatment of somatic disease, its unfavorable outcome; anxious fears (up to phobias) not connected with an actual somatic disease.

Negative affectivity is realized by phenomena of devitalization and mental alienation, which are maximally expressed at apathetic depression and are accompanied by awareness of change of own life activity. deep troubles. Negative affectivity includes the following psychopathological manifestations:

Painful insensitivity is the excruciating feeling of a loss of emotion, an inability to feel love, hate, compassion, or anger.

The phenomena of moral anesthesia - consciousness of mental discomfort with a sense of mental impoverishment, poverty of imagination, changes in emotional involvement with external objects, fading fantasy, loss of intuition, which previously allowed to unmistakably grasp the nuances of interpersonal relationships.

Depressive devitalization - feeling of weakening or disappearance of desire for life, instinct of self-preservation, somatosensory urges (sleep, appetite, libido).

Apathy is a deficiency of incentives with a loss of vitality, lethargy, indifference to everything around.

Dysphoria is gloomy sullenness, grumpiness, acrimony, grumpiness with complaints about others and demonstrative behavior.

Anguedonia - loss of the sense of pleasure, the ability to experience pleasure, love, joy, accompanied by the consciousness of inner dissatisfaction, mental discomfort[16].

In the current International Classification of Diseases - ICD-10 [34], which classifies mental and behavioral disorders according to the syndromic principle, the main importance is given to the correspondence of the clinical picture of the observed disorder to a set of standardized diagnostic criteria.

Within the Depressive Episode (F32), the main signs of depression are considered to be decreased mood, loss of interest and pleasure, decreased energy, which can lead to increased fatigue and decreased activity. Other symptoms of depression include decreased ability to concentrate and pay attention, decreased self-esteem, ideas of guilt and humiliation, pessimistic visions of the future, a tendency toward self-harm or suicide, sleep disturbances, and decreased appetite. The time factor is also given importance - the duration of a depressive episode is at least 2 weeks.

The ICD-10 classification of depressive disorders presented in Chapter V is very complex because of the multiplicity of diagnostic rubrics and their representation in the various sections. A total of 60 diagnostic rubrics must be used, subdivided as follows: affective (mood) disorders (F30-F39) - 40 rubrics; neurotic, stress-related and somatoform disorders (F40- F48) - 20 rubrics (including mixed anxiety-phobic disorders).

The ICD-10 diagnostic class "affective disorders" (F30-F39) comprises the categories: current depressive episode (F32), recurrent depression (F33), bipolar disorder with alternating depressive and manic phases (F31), and chronic mood disorders (F34), combining cyclothymia (F34.0) and dysthymia (F34.1). The Depressive Episode (major depression, unipolar or monopolar depression, and autonomic depression) occupies a central place in the systematics of affective pathology.

Among non-psychotic affective disorders of the ICD-10, but within the category "Neurotic, stress-related and somatoform disorders", "Mixed anxiety and depressive disorder" (F41.2) is placed under a separate heading. There are no clear diagnostic criteria for this disorder, which is observed mainly in the general medical network, in this classification. Only a general definition is given, according to which the condition in these cases corresponds to anxious depression (mild or unstable), characterized by a combination of anxious and depressive symptoms in the presence of at least some autonomic symptoms (e.g., tremor, palpitations, abdominal discomfort). Mixed anxiety and depressive disorder is diagnosed when these manifestations are relatively balanced.

Sleep disorders in the clinic of depression. Sleep is a functional state of the brain and the entire human organism with specific qualitative features of the central nervous system and somatic sphere activity that differ from wakefulness and are characterized by inhibition of active interaction of the organism with the environment and incomplete cessation of conscious mental activity. Sleep and wakefulness are functional states of a human, they are closely interconnected, and they should be considered in a single cycle [39].

Epidemiological studies show that about 35% of the population periodically suffers from insomnia. Any sleep disorders negatively affect human health, since sleep is the most important regulator of circadian (circadian) biological rhythms of the body, the significance of which lies in the regulation of organ and system function and interrelation with the external environment.

About 14% of patients seeking care from general practitioners complain of insomnia. Insomnia (insomnia) is a recurrent disorder of sleep initiation, duration, consolidation or quality that occurs despite the availability of sufficient time and conditions for sleep and is manifested by disturbances in daytime activity and activity. The DSM-IV defines insomnia as a deficit in the quality and quantity of nighttime sleep necessary for normal daytime activity. ICD-10 categorizes sleep disorders under F51, "Sleep disorders of inorganic nature", which describes dissomnia as a primarily psychogenic condition with an emotionally determined disorder of sleep quantity or time, i.e., insomnia, hypersomnia and sleep-wake cycle disorder.

Diagnostic criteria for sleep disorders include the presence of three or more of the following 7 signs, either continuously (more than a month) or periodically (more than three months): it takes more than 30 minutes to fall asleep; thoughts "creep into the head" all night; fear of being unable to fall asleep; frequent waking during the night; early waking and inability to go back to sleep; decreased mood and depression; unmotivated anxiety, fear.

According to the type of course in modern medicine, the following forms of insomnia are distinguished:

1) transient (transient), when sleep disturbances last from a few nights to several weeks;

2) periodic, when sleep is disrupted in certain life or seasonal cycles;

3) chronic, when sleep disturbances last for more than a month.

Sleep disorders are the most common in the clinic of depression and are among both its main and additional diagnostic criteria. The symptom complex of a depressive episode (according to ICD-10) includes not only hypothymia, anhedonia and decreased activity, fatigue and decreased self-esteem, but also ***early morning awakening (two hours or more before the usual wake-up time).***

Typology of depressive disorders. Vitality depression with the predominance of disorders of the positive affectivity circle belongs to the typical ones.

Vital depression in the clinic of affective disorders of *non-psychotic level* is usually defined by erased manifestations of melancholy with gratuitous pessimism, despondency, depression. In the picture of depression, melancholy, anxiety, guilt, and intellectual and motor inhibition are manifested. Unlike "psychotic depression", these disorders are not so persistent and prolonged. Feeling of homesickness can appear periodically throughout the day, but in the form of short episodes. In some cases, there can be overestimated ideas of shame and moral responsibility, but the lowered self-esteem does not reach the level of mastering ideas and coexists with competing ideas reflecting the real situation. Signs of idealizing inhibition may reach sufficient expression with a maximum in the morning hours, at the same time during the day a certain activity is preserved, the majority of patients continue to work, carry out (though with difficulty) their daily duties.

At *a psychotic level* of depression, brutal suicide attempts are possible. Melancholic depression at the psychotic level is characterized by a significant decrease in mood and pronounced ideational and motor lethargy. In patients, along with a depressed mood, an oppressive dystopia is noted. Vital melancholy is accompanied by oppressive, pressing sensations in the epigastrium, heaviness and pains in the heart. Everything is perceived in a gloomy light, and former grievances, misfortunes and wrong-doings resurface in memory and are overestimated. The present and future appear gloomy and hopeless. Patients spend whole days in a monotonous posture, sitting with their head low down, or lying in bed; their facial expressions are sorrowful and they have no desire for activity. Suicidal thoughts and tendencies testify to   the extreme severity of depression   [41,42,43,44].   Ideal retardation is manifested by slowed, quiet speech, difficulty processing new information, complaints of a sharp decrease in memory, and inability to concentrate.   The structure of melancholic depression is largely related   to the age of the patient at the time of its onset. The classic variation is characteristic of middle age. At a young age, the initial periods of these   depressions   are characterized by reflexivity, dysphoric disorders, and apathetic manifestations. These same patients develop typical melancholic depressions in adulthood.

Depending on their syndromic structure, sleep disorders have some specific features. From the point of view of modern views on clinical typology of depressions, V.N. Krasnov [45] singles out the following main variants: dreary-depressed, anxious-anxious and dreary-apathetic.

Mopey-loose depressions are among the true melancholic depressions in their traditional sense (46). They are characterized by a vitalization of the depressive affect with an unusually heavy, incomparable to everyday experience, wistful change of mood, up to intolerable pain, heaviness or burning in the chest, with lethargy and suppression of vital drives (libido, appetite). In these patients, the content of their experiences is defined by ideas of inferiority, self-deprecation, self-blaming and sometimes condemnation. Super-valuable and delusional ideas of hypochondriacal content are possible. Emotional disorders in boredom depressions also include anhedonia - absence of the habitual feeling of pleasure and mental anesthesia - "a sense of loss of feeling. Anesthesia of vital emotions is often manifested by a lack of a sense of sleep - a lack of a feeling of rest and vigor upon awakening, which is a frequent subject of complaints of these patients.

Thus, sleep disorders in wistful-lazy depressions are characterized by shortening of its duration and early morning awakening with deepening of depressed mood in the morning hours and experiences of "primary guilt" devoid of any explanation and ideational elaboration. In some patients, deterioration of mood and general well-being occurs after an afternoon nap.

Anxiety-anxiety depression is characterized by the prevalence in the clinical picture of depressive affect of feelings of inner restlessness, tension, which patients describe as a state of
"taut string inside", "clotting", "burning", etc. Anxiety experiences in these cases are characterized by constancy, shifting the greatest expression to a certain time of the day, not only to the morning hours, but also to the evening hours. Unlike dreary depressions accompanied with hypoesthesia, anxious depressions are characterized by hyperaesthesia - strengthening brightness of a sensual tone of perception. As a rule, perception of unpleasant and undesirable sensations (smells, sounds, etc.) which become irritating, aggravating the general depressed mood becomes acute. These patients become hypersensitive to previously insignificant psychologically traumatic situations with a long fixation on any emotionally negatively colored experiences which are characterized by a projection into the future of their presumed guilt, damage to others, expectation of an uncertain

trouble, misfortune or disaster.

Sleep disorders in anxious depression are mainly manifested by difficulty falling asleep, shallow sleep with frequent awakenings and nightmares. Patients complain about their inability to fall asleep because of a rush of unpleasant disturbing thoughts, fears that they will not be able to fall asleep, uncertain premonitions and fears. Restrictive behavior often develops in such patients. Patients anxiously wait for the night to come, are afraid to go to bed, are afraid to "die in their sleep", "fall asleep and do not wake up", or "have a nightmare night," which causes persistent insomnia. The main manifestation of this form of insomnia (psychophysiological insomnia) [45] is "fear of sleep", or rather fear of not falling asleep again. A negative association is gradually formed when the very thought of having to go to bed leads to brain activation. Persistent sleep disorders significantly worsen not only the mental but also the somatic state of these patients.

Dreary-apathetic depressions are characterized by a combination of depressed mood and a lack of motivation for activity. In these patients, apathy develops as motivational depression within the limits of the affective disorder proper, i.e. with experience of lack of interest in any or weakly significant activity. These patients are characterized by an increase in withdrawal, detachment, and narrowing of interests and socialization. Sleep disorders in boredom-apathic depressions most often take the form of hypersomnia. Sufficiently long night's sleep does not bring these patients the desired alertness, and general lethargy and somnolence remain throughout the day, but they can also complain about a complete lack of sleep for many nights, which is a manifestation of pseudoinsomnia. The main symptom-forming factor in this case is impaired perception of one's own sleep, related to the peculiarities of the sense of time at night due to depression. However, on objective polysomnographic examination, sleep is not only present, but its duration exceeds 8 hours (distorted sleep perception or "sleep agnosia ", "sleep hypochondria "). Because of persistent sleep disturbances, such Patients are often unable to work properly and become a burden to their loved ones.

Atypical depression. In the literature, atypical depression is defined as depression in which the clinical picture contains phenomena of depersonalization, derealization, senesto- hypochondriacal disorders, paranoid formations, sensory delirium, delirium inclusions. At the same time, the affects of melancholy, apathy, anxiety, circadian-vital components are relegated to the background or completely masked. The increase in the number of patients with atypical and insufficiently differentiated forms of depression is often associated with the phenomena of drug pathomorphosis and, in particular, on the one hand, the transition of many mental disorders to the circadian level, and on the other hand, with an increase in the number of cases of prolonged, incurable, sterile, "matte" forms of depression with poor and low-mobile symptoms [47,48,49].

In these cases, phobias, anxieties, hypochondria are observed instead of the typical vital longing, mental pain, and vital worries can take on a bizarre character in the form of increasing somatic complaints in the morning ("stomach discomfort", heaviness or pain in the head, "body numbness", "lack of air", unpleasant sensations in the heart area, etc.). Instead of motor retardation, there may be fidgetiness, "constant rushing," and instead of slowed intellectual activity, there may be difficulties in making decisions, ambivalence, and impaired concentration.

Cerebral, vascular, somatic, and endocrine pathology is traditionally believed to be involved in the formation of atypical depression. In milder states, apathy is introduced into the clinical picture due to premorbid psychopathological features, reactive moments, somato-vegetative symptoms. Quite often atypical depression is observed in adolescence or late adulthood. In this case, depression often manifests as behavioral disorders (delinquent behavior) or in the form of numerous, often unusual somatic complaints[13, 49].

Atypical depression with predominance of negative affectivity. The clinical picture of *apathetic depression* is dominated by a deficit of motivations and a decrease in vital tonus. All of the patients' acts as though lose internal sense, are committed by virtue of necessity, "out of habit,
"automatically." Apathetic affect is associated with impoverishment of facial expressions, monotony of speech, slowness of movements. Depression is manifested by a sudden feeling of detachment from previous desires, indifference to one's surroundings and own situation, lack of interest in the results of one's own activities. The changed feeling sharply contrasts with the pre-depression feeling. In the foreground (though under the mask of indifference or inactivity to events in one's environment), there is a gloomy depression associated with awareness of the changes in one's affective life ("syndrome of loss"). The following types of apathetic degression are distinguished:

Adynamic depression is characterized by a loss of initiative and impulse to spontaneous activity. The clinical picture is dominated by motor lethargy, adynamy, up to the degree of spontaneity, stupor, weakness, lethargy, impotence, impossibility or difficulty to perform physical or mental *work while the urges, desires and desire for activity remain.* Ideal, motor and a combined version of these depressions are distinguished.

In the ideational variant, the adynamic symptoms prevail over depression proper. Mood is lowered, patients express ideas of inferiority, but the basic plot of experiences consists of adynamic disorders. Adynamy is expressed in complaints about the absence of
"moral strength", "mental impotence", poor judgment. In the depressive triad, ideatorial inhibition dominates over motor inhibition.

The motor variant of adynamic depressions is characterized by the prevalence of a feeling of powerlessness, brokenness, lethargy and muscular relaxation. The affective radical is represented by depression with a sense of inner restlessness and tension. In the depressive triad, motor lethargy predominates over ideational lethargy. Somatic signs of depression (sleep disturbances, appetite, libido, weight loss) are distinctly expressed. Delusions of own inferiority, the contents of which are defined by features of adynamy, are noted[50].<u>The combined</u> variant of depression is characterized by the phenomena of both motor and ideational adynamy. Anxiety and melancholy of uncertain nature are present. Motor retardation prevails in the depressive triad. Self-image of inferiority is accompanied by a feeling of self-pity. Severe somatic disorders are noted.

Asthenic depression (depression of exhaustion, neurasthenic melancholy). Asthenia is one of the symptom-forming manifestations of depression. In some cases, it acts as a prodromal affective disorder[51]. The picture of an unfolded asthenic depression includes increased exhaustion, decreased activity, weakness, complaints of physical impotence, loss of energy, "weariness". Any activity is associated with overcoming infirmity and is not satisfying. A feeling of fatigue occurs with little effort. In patients with mild depression, functioning can be preserved and is accompanied by increased exhaustion. *An abnormal circadian rhythm is characteristic.* The feature of depressive fatigue that distinguishes it from ordinary fatigue is a special feeling of muscle lethargy and impairment of the general sense of body. Depressive asthenia is characterized by persistence and lack of connection with workload. With a more pronounced depressive affect, the complaints of difficulties even in performing the usual morning procedures (washing, dressing) are characteristic. The latter are exhausting and take much longer than usual. There are signs of irritable weakness and hyperesthesia. Affective displays are limited, sadness, anxiety and ideas of worthlessness are not typical. Pessimism with a sense of hopelessness, depression and indifference prevails. More often asthenic depressions are somatogenic (symptomatic), arising at severe chronic somatic (diabetes, anemia, liver cirrhosis) and neurological diseases (atherosclerosis of cerebral vessels, multiple sclerosis, Parkinson's disease) [52].

Anesthetic (depersonalization) depression is defined by a phenomenon of alienation of emotions, which extends to both interpersonal relations and phenomena of the external world. What is going on around does not resonate in the soul, everything seems altered, unnatural, alien.In mild versions of depression, alienation is manifested by a muted sensation. The feeling of change of emotional belonging to the outside world, "existence behind a barrier" dominates. Self-awareness disorders proceed with a picture of moral anesthesia. The phenomena of painful alienation are manifested by the consciousness of dissatisfaction with one's own mental activity, "moral ugliness" due to deautomatization of mental functions, loss of the ability to establish consistent connections between events, assimilation of the elementary meaning of things. Although the level of alienation is relatively shallow and manifests itself mainly in a decrease in the saturation of perception and imagination, fears of irreversibility of changes in mental activity, constant comparison with previous, pre-moral abilities are brought to the fore. Symptom complexes of moral anesthesia are not stable and are completely reduced as depression develops inversely. Alienation phenomena are usually accompanied by anhedonia with loss of feeling of pleasure, ability to rejoice, to experience pleasure.

Depression with alienation of somatosensory cravings is limited to the manifestations of the somatic sphere - sudden loss of the need for sleep, satiation (depressive anorexia), reduction, up to complete disappearance of the sexual desire. Sleep disorders, as well as the reduction of hunger, have a total character. Aversion to food is accompanied by refusal to eat and malnutrition with significant weight loss over the course of 1-2 weeks of the disease. Pathological circadian rhythm and depressive mood are present, with manifestations of pathologically reduced affect limited to sterile hypothymia.The somatic equivalents of depression with alienation of somatosensory drives can precede the manifestation of affective disorders of other types (vital, hypochondriacal depression). The latter occur either as psychopathological manifestations deepen in the present or in subsequent phases of the illness[11,13].

Depressions formed by accentuation of one of the obligate components of the affective syndrome.

Anxiety depression. In the clinical picture, along with depression, psychiatric or somatic, accompanied by massive somatovegetative disorders, manifestations of anxiety predominate. Patients are fearful, depressed, depressed.In some cases, in the foreground is internal tension, uncertain anxiety ("a vague threat hangs in the air", "something must happen"), sometimes felt physically as internal trembling, and not finding specific reasons and explanations (vital, free-floating, generalized anxiety). Fears of an imagined or hypertrophied threatening misfortune, uncertainty about the future, fear of unexpected, unforeseen events ("forward anxiety"), or anxious doubts about the timeliness or legitimacy of acts already performed, the validity of what is said with a set of self-reproaches ("backward anxiety") can dominate. Sometimes the clinic is defined by doubts about the possibility of making the simplest everyday decisions, manifested in indecision, uncertainty in one's actions in the present ("lunacy of doubts") [11,32,53].Anxiety is often found in patients with endogenous depression. Many authors are convinced that depression always proceeds with anxiety. Moreover, it is impossible to differentiate between depression and anxiety on the basis of psychopathological features[54,55].The distinction between anxiety and depression could not be made in the pharmacological experiment either, because the anxiety affect
The depressive mood "takes" with it a part of the depressive mood. Such close coexistence of the affects of melancholy and anxiety complicates their differentiation and is the reason that in depression, it is almost always possible to find elements of anxiety and tension, and the state of anxiety is characterized by a lowered mood.The dominant affect determines the nature of the pathologically altered mood, but does not exclude the presence of other affects. In case of prevalence of melancholy affects, the mood is evaluated as depressive, in case of prevalence of anxiety - as anxious; when both affective components are significantly expressed, the syndrome is evaluated as anxious-depressive, and exact evaluation of mood as a symptom becomes difficult.

Anxiety-depressive syndrome may cause melancholy with a vital component, a pathological circadian rhythm. In the motor sphere, there can be either motor restlessness, up to and including abrupt agitation, or anxious stupor, up to and including immobility. Depressive ideas can have a dual nature ("guilty, but I am afraid of punishment") and hypochondriacal ideas are frequent. If there are obsessions, they have a phobic character. Depersonalizing phenomena are possible. In addition to reduction of appetite and constipation, muscle cramps and painful sensations are also noted, which quite often serve as a basis for hypochondriacal experiences. The risk of suicide is very high. Suicide attempts often have an impulsive character. Patients with postpartum, somatoform and involutionary depression are especially dangerous in this respect. Extended suicides are possible[56,57].

Self-torturing depression is defined by the prevalence of negative self-esteem, ideas of inferiority and guilt.

Gradually, as depression develops, these ideas acquire the character of dominating or super-valuable. The feeling of shame often comes to the foreground, being a source of constant self-representations: for as if unworthy behavior in the past, for a wrongly lived life, the broken moral standards, etc. Ideas of guilt or sinfulness may acquire the most persistent character. In cases where the meaningful complex of depression is formed on the background of relatively reduced affective disorders, the concept of self-blame tends to systematize and transform into depressive delirium (57).

Hypochondriacal depression. Hypothymia is combined with anxious fears about one's health, hypochondriacal phobias, and somatovegetative disorders. There is a pessimistic perception of real or imagined somatic pathology and a hypertrophied assessment of its consequences.

The dominant perceptions are about the danger (usually exaggerated) of internal organ dysfunctions that manifest the disease process, its unfavorable outcome, and the futility of treatment. In the foreground:
- fear of the onset or exacerbation of a tumor process
  or other serious illness;
- Fear of death from a sudden heart attack,often accompanied by panic
  attacks;
- fear of being in a situation that excludes the possibility of medical
  help, agoraphobia;
- phenomena of acute self-observation with careful registration of the
  slightest signs of bodily malaise.

Among somatovegetative manifestations, sleep disturbances (especially its continuity with "disconnected sleep" in the second half of the night and early awakening) prevail. Worsening of well-being in the morning hours, feeling unrefreshed in the head, appetite disorder, vasomotor disorders are present, accompanied by copious somatopsychic complaints (feeling of somatic malaise, tightness and heaviness in the chest, volatile joint pains, chills, etc.). Hypochondriacal depression is not uncommon in general medical practice. In an effort to verify their fears, patients go to internists first, insisting on multiple examinations.

Dysphoric depression is a condition characterized by the occurrence of dysphoria, i.e. irritability, anger, aggression and destructive tendencies against a background of low mood. At the same time, objects and situations which have not recently attracted attention can suddenly become a source of irritation. The behavior of patients can be various: some patients have a predominance of aggression and threats to others, destructive tendencies; others have a desire for solitude connected with hyperesthesia and "hatred of the world"; others have a desire for activity which is not directed. At the moment of development of dysphoria sometimes the sensation of internal mental tension with expectation of the approaching disaster prevails[32].

Depressions formed due to the accession of psychopathological manifestations of non-affective registers.

Depression with obsessions (complicated depression): the clinical picture is dominated by obsessions that converge in the structure of affective disorders. Obsessive-phobic disorders that form as part of depression are represented by anxiety fears, obsessive ideas of worthlessness and self-blame, obsessive suicidal thoughts. Panic attacks are also observed, with massive somatovegetative and conversion symptoms, as well as phobias of hypochondriacal content.Within the limits of anxious depressions, contrast obsessions - fears of loss of control over oneself, a possibility to commit self-destructive, socially-unacceptable and criminal acts can manifest. As anxiety and internal tension builds up, there is a fear of inflicting serious and even lethal damage on oneself or others.

Hysterical depression. The clinical picture is characterized by a particular brightness of symptoms, often combined with other hysterical manifestations - pseudodenation, puerilism, delusional fantasies. Hysterical "stigmata" in the form of paresias, aphonias, blepharospasm, etc. are also observed. The affect of melancholy is unstable and shallow, and is combined with irritability, dissatisfaction and moodiness. Psychomotor retardation is usually absent or expressed insignificantly. More often, such conditions arise in response to the breakup of a love relationship or death of loved ones. In these cases, hysterical depression proceeds with a picture of a pathological reaction of grief. Dissociative disorders with sensation of physical presence of a close person who has become a victim of catastrophe, "dialogue" with him or her acquiring the form of dialogue dominate. Manifestations of depression are combined with features of theatricality and deliberateness. Memories of tragedy have a character of overwhelming representations, are accompanied by weeping with tears, groans, wringing of hands and fainting. The desire to draw the attention of others to one's grief is quite often accompanied by demonstrative self-destructive displays (superficial cuts, scratches, etc.) with threats or even attempts at suicide. Patients may assert that other people's grief is nothing in comparison with their suffering and that those around them underestimate their distress. Sometimes depression becomes agitated, but even in these cases, facial, vasodilatory and motor expressions remain as expressive. Self-repression, if it occurs, gives the impression of being deliberate and unnatural, usually, the tendency to blame others, rather than oneself, for one's misfortunes is noted and quite often exaggerated concerns about one's health are expressed. Psychogenichallucinations are complex, complex, often playing out in the sphere of several sense organs. The sharp discrepancy between the massiveness of manifestations of hysterical depression and the comparatively small disadaptation of patients attracts attention. If necessary in the family or office environment, they can "switch over," "pull themselves together" and cope with all current affairs.

Depression with delirium. Delusional symptom complexes combined with depression include both depressive delirium and more complex psychopathological entities.Depressive delirium is more often limited to typical themes of shame ("paranoia of conscience"), guilt (delirium of sinfulness, self-blame, somatic illness (hypochondriac delirium)). In presenting the clinical picture, there is a tendency for expansion of paranoid manifestations: along with delusions of guilty conscience and self-blame, there are ideas of attitude, delusions of condemnation and accusation. Anxiety and fear increase. Patients "notice" the judgmental glances of others, expect imminent punishment.Delusional depressions are characterized by high levels of anxiety, persistent sleep disorders, psychomotor agitation; the risk of suicidal behavior is very high. Delusional depressions are most common in involuticnary melancholia, schizoaffective psychosis, and schizophrenia.

Depressive state with delirium and hallucinations. Catatonic disorders can occupy a large place in the structure of these depressions - from separate manifestations in the form of an increase in muscle tone, negativism, to pronounced pictures of stupor and substupor.In the existing classifications, besides those described above, there are often tearful, ironic, stupor depression, etc. But the characteristics reflected in the names of these depressions are not essential. But the characteristics reflected in the names of these depressions are not essential. They only emphasize certain characteristics of the depressive state, which can be observed in the picture of depressions of different structures[11,32].

Masked depression is also referred to as "hidden" depression,
The latter are either "lauric", "alexithymic depressions", or as "thymopathic (depressive) equivalents". In all these cases, we are talking about subdepressive states combined with expressed, and often dominating in the clinical picture, vegetative-somatic disorders. Their intensity in comparison with a slightly lowered mood, which is more or less obscured, allows to designate such kind of depression as latent. The frequency of such hidden depressions, encountered almost, if not exclusively, in outpatient practice, exceeds the number of obvious depressions by 10-20 times. Such patients are initially treated by physicians of various specialties, most often general practitioners and neurologists, and are admitted for psychiatric observation (if at all), often long after the onset of the illness.

The symptomatology of such latent depressions is extremely diverse. The most frequent are complaints of disorders of the cardiovascular system and digestive organs: short-term, prolonged, often in the form of paroxysms, pain in the heart area, accompanied in some cases by irradiation of pain, as in angina pectoris; various disorders of heart rhythm, up to paroxysms of atrial fibrillation, variations in blood pressure levels; reduced appetite, up to and including anorexia, diarrhea, constipation, flatulence, pain along the gastrointestinal tract, etc.д. Pathological, particularly painful sensations are very common: neuralgic paresthesias, migrating or localized pains (pain characteristic of lumbago, toothache, headaches). Disorders resembling bronchial asthma and diencephalic paroxysms occur. Various sleep disorders are very often observed. Due to the fact that depressive disorders are difficult to identify, but connection of somatic disorders with depression is undoubted, many people call autonomic-somatic disorders found in latent depression depressive equivalents. The number of such equivalents has been increasing over the years. Comparing the psychopathology of hidden depression to the onset of depression in general, the similarity between it and the somatic component is hard to miss. It's possible that hidden depression is an initial stage in the development of depression in which there is no deepening of mental disorders for a long time, and the somatic symptoms are distinct. This suggestion is supported by cases of prolonged silent depression, in which a distinct depressive component finally emerges 3-5 years after onset, and by those cases in which the illness develops intermittently and again years later deteriorates into both somatic and overt depressive disorders. Positive results of therapy with antidepressants also testify to the mental conditioning of somatic disorders.There are several variants of masked depression (Appendix 1)Depressions that take on somatic "masks" are more common in the general medical network. According to S. Lesse. between 1 in 3 and 2 in 3 of all patients seen by general practitioners suffer from masked depression. It is not uncommon for manifestations of depression to overlap with algic symptoms (ICD-10 section F45.4-Cronic Somatoform Pain Disorder). This disorder has a high comorbidity with depression (60-100%), suggesting that it may represent a variant of masked depression, but it cannot be excluded that in these cases, depression may be a consequence of chronic pain syndrome[58,59]. Many psychiatrists present a narrower definition of masked depression, referring only to somatized forms of endogenous depression (32). The psychopathological picture of these conditions is close to the hypochondriacal depression, but it is accompanied by distinctly expressed somato-vegetative disorders in the foreground. These disorders could be classified as depressions, depending on their phases, their distinctive circadian rhythm, a hereditary burden of affective illnesses, the presence of more typical affective phases in the anamnesis, and good efficacy of thymoanaleptic therapy. Masked depression is not a clinical diagnosis, much less a nosological one, because both endogenous and psychogenic depression can hide behind a somatic mask. Masked depression is a clinical term indicating that, phenomenologically, these conditions are close to depression, although they are temporarily dominated by somatic symptoms that have no real organic basis.

3. Pathogenetic patterns of anxiety and diagnosis of anxiety disorders

Psychologically normal anxiety, according to R. D. Levitov (1969), is a psychological state caused by possible or probable unpleasantness, uncertainty, changes in the habitual situation and activity, a delay of pleasant, desirable things and expressed in specific experiences (fears, worries, disturbances of peace) and reactions.

Normal anxiety prepares the individual for a protective response, and the sympathetic department of the autonomic nervous system becomes active: heart rate and cardiac output increase, bronchial smooth muscle tone decreases, respiratory rate and depth increase, metabolic processes increase, thus preparing the body for activity. This level of anxiety allows you to cope with an unpleasant situation.

High levels of anxiety have a debilitating and even disorganizing effect on the human psyche. *Anxiety goes beyond the norm* when its intensity and duration are disproportionate to the possible damage, and also when it occurs in a neutral situation or in a situation containing no objective threat. Both the acute short-term stress reaction and the longer-term stress state have a strong impact on the occurrence and course of most illnesses.

Personal anxiety is interpreted as a stable tendency of a particular person to perceive and evaluate a wide range of phenomena as carrying potential danger. Anxiety, as a characteristic feature, increases with age, which is caused by biological processes of involution and the reaction of an aging person to a new situation developed under the influence of biological and social factors.

Neurotic anxiety can be outwardly gratuitous "free-floating" as well as closely related to phobias and obsessions, somatopsychic sensations and senestopathies.

Psychotic anxiety is traditionally described within the framework of manic-depressive psychosis (bipolar affective disorder), schizophrenia, involutional and vascular psychoses. Psychotic anxiety is a nonspecific compensatory response to a disturbance of certain brain structures or a result of a disturbance of the functional systems involved in the genesis of anxiety.

The range of manifestations of anxiety is very wide and extends from mild, barely noticeable reactions in the structure of the personality to developed psychopathological conditions requiring treatment in an inpatient setting. Anxiety can manifest as part of non-psychotic states, reactions, psychogenias, somatogenias and also in the structure of endogenous psychoses. The universal and, therefore, nonspecific nature of anxiety affect causes difficulties in differential diagnosis, requiring clinicians to carefully distinguish anxiety from other similar affective disorders. Anxiety refers to the symptomatology of internal tension and anxiety with presentiment of threat and pessimistic apprehension. Psychopathological symptoms of anxiety can be difficult to verbalize, especially for patients with alexithymia. The most typical are complaints of an excruciating feeling of constraint and a feeling of helplessness in the face of some uncertain threat. Anxiety must be differentiated from fear, which, unlike anxiety, has a concrete content and object, i.e., it arises in relation to a definite threat; fear does not affect the essence of the personality and the personality retains its internal resources[60,61].

Pathogenetic regularities of anxiety. From the point of view of modern concepts the emergence and regulation of anxiety is provided by a complex interaction of several mediator systems: catecholaminergic, serotoninergic, endocrine, etc. The interaction between excitatory amines (glutamate, aspartate) and the GABAergic system is the most important for the regulation of neuronal activity. A shift in the balance towards the excitatory amines leads to an increase in neuronal activity (increase in alertness), the occurrence of anxiety, agitation, insomnia. Obviously, none of the systems, taken separately, can be responsible for the manifestation of anxiety. Anxiety should be seen as the end result of the interaction of a variety of biochemical factors. Because several endogenous neuroactive metabolites are involved in the genesis of anxiety, there are a number of hypotheses for its neurochemical support. [62].

The catecholamine hypothesis is based on the finding that anxiety states are associated with increased levels of catecholamines (especially adrenaline) in the urine, with the central release of these substances preceding their peripheral release by the adrenal glands. Of great importance here is the disruption of the function of the so-called "blue spot" (Locus coeruleus). The latter is a small nucleus in the brainstem containing approximately 50% of all noradrenergic neurons of the CNS.

Stimulation of the "blue spot" leads to sympathetic excitation and release of catecholamines, which is symptomatically manifested as a panic attack. Catecholamine activators, such as adrenaline, amphetamine, and caffeine, also have a distinct anxiolytic effect.

The hypothesis related to benzodiazepine receptors that regulate GABA metabolism is based on the fact that GABA is the brain's main neurotransmitter; it opens the ion channels of nerve cell membranes, reducing their excitability and reducing anxiety. It is believed that patients with anxiety disorders secrete metabolites that block these receptors, leading to anxiety. A possible cause of anxiety may also be insufficient activity of the GABAergic system, particularly the GABA-benzodiazepine receptor complex [63].

The serotonin hypothesis was introduced into the neurochemistry of affective disorders in 1969. Subsequently, the effect of serotonergic antidepressants in some anxiety disorders led to the assumption of a role of serotonin balance in the appearance of anxiety. It has been suggested that prolonged anxiety arousal leads to the release of serotonin and the formation of a pathological feedback formed by a compensatory decrease in the number of presynaptic 5NT1a receptors. The latter leads to increased discharge by serotonin neurons and additional serotonin release. Therefore, serotonin-positive agents (IMAOs, serotonin reuptake inhibitors, etc.), causing even greater stimulation of neurons, can provoke aggravation of anxiety, but later such powerful activation leads to desensitization of these receptors with loss of their sensitivity to the transmitter. The impulse activity of the neuron and the release of serotonin are normalized.Thus, an evolutionary system of multilink neurochemical support of anxiety as a universal reaction of the organism aimed at implementation of resistance and escape was formed.The adaptive role of anxiety in animals was described by W. B. Cannon (1929), describing it as a "fight and flight reaction". This reaction is characterized by a number of physiological shifts that prepare the body for a rapid response to danger: the release of adrenaline increases, the sympathetic system is activated, resulting in increased blood pressure, increased blood flow in the muscles and brain, blood glucose levels increase to create the most favorable conditions for these systems to function. Increase of blood clotting protects from great blood loss in case of wound, increase of glucocorticoids secretion protects from acute anaphylactic reaction when foreign substances get into wounds. These and other physiological shifts have a distinct adaptive character, but if they are too strong and prolonged, they may also be the cause of somatic catastrophes and diseases: heart attack, stroke, hypertensive crisis, later - diabetes, hypertension, etc. [64].G.Selye (1936) extended the data of W. B. Cannon with the concept of stress (nonspecific adaptation syndrome). The latter refers mainly to the involvement of the endocrine system in the reactions to extreme situations. Anxiety itself, taking into account the nature of neuroendocrine reactions, can be defined as a mental component of stress. The term "anxiety' is also used to denote a complex of biochemical, endocrine, neurovegetative and mental processes in the first stage of stress. Depending on the initial situation of the body, the adaptation syndrome proceeds differently. It is conventionally accepted that at the stage of anxiety there is a mobilization of the available functional reserves. The adaptation phase is characterized by the destruction of the old and formation of the new

The "functional systemicity" adequate to the extreme requirements of the environment and the steady expenditure of the adaptation resources. In the exhaustion phase there is a breakdown of regulatory mechanisms with irreversible somatic changes[65].Thus, the above historical and modern concepts of etiopathogenesis of anxiety disorders provide an opportunity to choose and justify the medical tactics in each specific case - to build an adequate clinical model of the disease, stages of examination and therapy, implementation of interdisciplinary principle of patient management, taking into account competence of allied specialists.

Diagnosis of anxiety disorders. The main method for diagnosing anxiety disorders is clinical and psychopathological, which includes collecting and analyzing anamnestic information about the patient, and describing his or her mental status.

In 1909 E. Kraepelin was one of the first to describe anxiety in detail on the pages of the 8th edition of his manual: "If a painful mournful tone is accompanied by a feeling of inner tension, the mental mood acquires the character of anxiety (Aengstlichkeit). The patient loses his inner confidence and sense of freedom, his confidence in his own strength and abilities. Each action is followed by painful expectations of its consequences, doubts about its correctness and expediency. Here, too, the state of one's own body provides particularly fertile ground for all kinds of fears, and the result is painful self-pity, wisecracks, and a heightened sense of responsibility; they drown out in the end the timid impulses of self-confident vigor. This tone of emotion serves as the basis on which obsessive perceptions, compulsive fears, and the neurosis of expectation especially often develop." Anxiety (Angst), which E. Kraepelin regarded as a combination of a feeling of discontent with inner tension, he considered the most common form of pathological emotion. "No feeling affects the spiritual and physical condition so much as this. The inner tension is found in the posture of the body, the expressive movements, the convulsive inertia of the muscles, or it is discharged in yelling and screaming, in violent attempts at defense and flight, in attempts on others or on one's own life. To this are joined all the nervous phenomena accompanying anxiety, known from normal life: dizziness, nausea, a feeling of relaxation, action on heart activity (palpitation), on the nerves of the vessels (pallor, increased blood pressure), on breathing, on the voluntary muscles (trembling, staggering), finally, on perspiration, on emptying the bladder and rectum. The effects on breathing and cardiac activity are perceived very vividly by the patients, as a feeling of tightness in the cardiac region." "At the beginning the feeling of anxiety is, as a rule, unpremeditated; the patient feels it without knowing why, often even realizing quite clearly that he has nothing to fear... Of course vague anxious premonitions are usually gradually connected with more or less clearly outlined apprehensions. In the higher stages of anxiety, consciousness is more or less obscured; very strong mental excitement allows only completely vague and confused perceptions." The variety of symptom complexes accompanying anxiety makes it much more difficult to identify, so the clinical and psychopathological examination of the patient should pay attention to the combination of the four main components of anxiety: affective, ideational, motor and autonomic[63].

The ***affective component of anxiety*** is manifested by feelings of gratuitous excitement and anxiety, vague premonitions and fearful expectations of impending trouble. Increased irritability, emotional intemperance, feelings of agitation and being "on the edge of a breakdown" are usually accompanied by sleep disorders in the form of difficulty falling asleep, shallow sleep and unpleasant dreams.

Ideator symptoms of anxiety include signs of accelerated thinking (up to and including an anxious feeling of incomplete thought control), as well as a tendency to anxious thoughts, absent-mindedness, and difficulty concentrating. There can be both "forward anxiety" - heavy premonitions in connection with insignificant excuses, and "backward anxiety" - unjustified anxiety about the possible mistakes made or in connection with the already happened events, which negative consequences are exaggerated. The content of anxiety anxiety is defined not so much by situational moments, but by individually significant catatymic complexes.

The motor component of anxiety is manifested by a feeling of special muscular discomfort, which is perceived by patients as internal tension. At the same time, patients complain of a feeling of "tightness", "compression" in the chest, headaches, muscle pain, back and lower back pain, muscle twitching, inner trembling, fidgeting. Outwardly stiff patients note an "inability to relax", "inner tension" accompanied by a feeling of physical weakness and muscle fatigue.

The vegetative component of anxiety is manifested by a wide range of somatovegetative sensations: sweating, discomfort in the epigastric region, dry mouth, dizziness, unsteadiness when walking, shortness of breath, difficulty breathing, heart pain, palpitations, chills, hot or cold waves, numbness in hands and feet, whose severity correlates with the level of emotional tension manifested by anxiety.

The criteria by which to distinguish true somatic disorders from signs of somatization of anxiety and depression are important for general clinical practitioners:

1. Lack of objective signs of somatic disease or disproportionality of severe subjective sensations of the patient to objectively detected somatic pathology;

2. Inconsistency of the somatovegetative "facade" with the clinical picture of the somatic disease, even taking into account the individual variability of its manifestations;

3. Migration of symptoms of somatic suffering (change of complaints from one organ system to another);

4. Presence of stable pathogenetically unreasonable variants of a combination of somatovegetative symptoms of different functional systems;

5. Specific medical history:

-uncertainty in the diagnosis of somatic suffering (type of "dystonia," "dysfunction," etc.);

-unconfirmed by objective methods of diagnosis of somatic disease;

persistence in seeking medical help, despite the apparent lack of results of treatment;

-ineffectiveness of somatic therapy.

The classification of anxiety disorders given in ICD-10 (1994) is as follows: Anxiety-phobic disorders (agoraphobia, social phobia, isolated (specific) phobia, other and unspecified phobic disorders); other anxiety disorders (panic disorder, generalized anxiety, mixed anxiety-depression, other specified and unspecified anxiety disorders); obsessive-compulsive disorder, reactions to severe stress and adaptive disorders including. including post-traumatic stress disorder.

Generalized anxiety disorder (GAD), adjustment disorder, and mixed anxiety-depressive disorder are among the most frequently encountered anxiety conditions in psychiatric and general clinical practice.

The Basic Principles of Therapy for Depression

Before prescribing a therapeutic program, a thorough examination of the patient with the collection of subjective and objective information about his condition, dominant symptomatology, its duration and connection with possible psychotraumatic situations, assessment of the degree of suicidal risk is necessary. It is necessary to analyze the features of the course of the disease, hereditary aggravation of mental disorders of the affective spectrum, the nature of therapy and the reaction to it in previous exacerbations.

Immediately after the establishment of even a preliminary diagnosis of depression, it is necessary to make *a plan of therapeutic measures*, which should include the following tasks:

1) Rapid relief of acute depressive symptoms in order to reduce the patient's suffering and prevent suicide;
2) Complete elimination of depressive symptoms, stabilization of the condition and achievement of remission;
3) Restoration of the previous level of psychological, social and labor adaptation (psychotherapeutic and social rehabilitation);
4) Preventing or reducing the risk of developing an exacerbation or new episode.

The choice of the antitussive and thymoanaleptic therapy (ATT), its intensity should be based on nosological and syndromological diagnosis of depression and severity of its symptomatology.

TAT is primarily needed for endogenous depression with a unipolar or bipolar course. For depressive symptoms developing in schizoaffective disorder (SAD) and schizophrenia, TAT should be combined with neuroleptics. Somatogenic depression requires pathogenetic somatic therapy and only secondarily symptomatic psychopharmacotherapy. Dysthymic disorders and situational (reactive) depressions of a neurotic level are treated quite well both with antidepressants and certain kinds of psychotherapy.

It is necessary to understand that any depression is a *complex psychosomatic phenomenon, mediated by the personality* of the patient and needs a complex pharmacotherapy, psychotherapy and somatic treatment.

The decisive factor for prescribing a particular antidepressant is the *exact qualification of the leading psychopathological syndrome*. Antidepressants with a sedative effect are used for anxious forms of depression, with a stimulating (activating) effect - for lethargic (apato-anergic) forms of depression   .Figure 2 illustrates the criteria antidepressants for depression with positive affectivity phenomena.

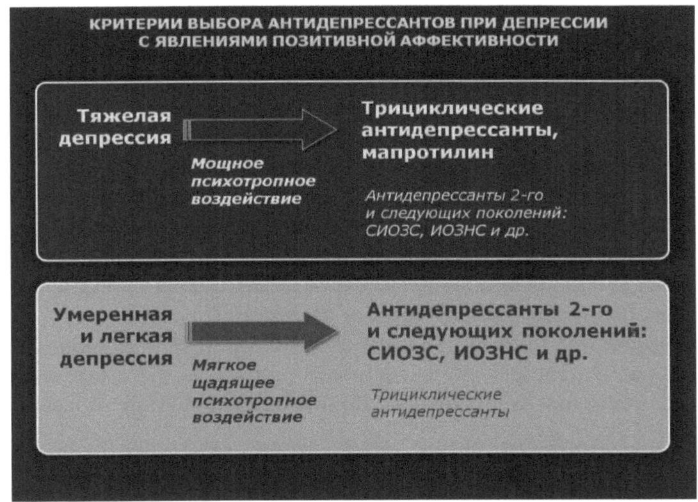

Figure 2 - Selection Criteria for Antidepressants

The general rule for most tricyclic antidepressants is that therapy is started with 25 to 50 mg/day and within 3 to 4 days, doses are brought up to therapeutically effective. If there is good tolerance and no effect within 10 days, half the maximum dose (for tricyclic antidepressants it is about 150 mg/day) is quickly raised to the maximum dose (250 to 300 mg/day). When used for serotonergic antidepressants, the dose is fixed immediately for the duration of therapy. The dosage does not change even with subsequent prolonged prophylactic therapy. However, in some cases (with individual sensitivity to the drug), it is reasonable to prescribe treatment with minimal doses of serotonergic antidepressants. Many patients respond more effectively to lower doses of medication. When selecting an adequate dose of serotonergic antidepressants, it is possible to be guided in part by the side effects that occur: nausea in the first week of therapy, drowsiness after an equilibrium concentration is established after 2-3 weeks of treatment. The therapeutic effect often develops more gradually than with tricyclic antidepressants, therefore it is not recommended to change the dose for 4 - 8 weeks. Usually clinical effect of antidepressants develops in 2-3 weeks after their application in adequate doses. Drugs with a sedative effect are used mainly at night, and with a stimulating effect in the morning and during the day. Differential use of tricyclic antidepressants at different times of the day (imipramine in the morning, and amitriptyline in the evening), taking into account the syndrome variant (anxious or melancholic) has rapid (8-10 days of treatment)

therapeutic effect in most patients with endogenous depression. To increase the therapeutic effect of antidepressants and to correct the side effects of thymoleptic agents in the treatment of endogenous depression, Magnes B 6 is used.

In the absence of any effect after 3-4 weeks, it is necessary to switch to another antidepressant, preferably of a different chemical structure and a different mechanism of action. If there is some relief, especially with serotonergic antidepressants, it is more reasonable to continue therapy for up to 6-8 weeks, as the effect in many patients develops gradually. The main criterion for changing drugs after 3-4 weeks is a complete absence of reduction of depressive symptoms. If there is at least a small progressive improvement at optimal doses, wait for a more pronounced effect after 8-12 weeks.

In a holistic approach to the treatment of depression as a chronic recurrent illness, we can distinguish *3 main stages of therapy*:

1) The *suppressive therapy* is aimed at rapid relief of symptoms from the beginning of treatment of the depressive phase to the establishment of clinical remission. With adequate thymoanaleptic therapy, it lasts 6 to 12 weeks.

2) *The finalizing therapy* consists of the continuation of taking an effective antidepressant from the moment of achieving clinical (therapeutic) remission until the supposed spontaneous end of the phase. The duration of this phase varies widely and depends on the endogenously programmed characteristics of the disease - with a unipolar course it is usually 5-9 months, and with a bipolar course - 3-4 months, as the risk of phase inversion and development of an unfavorable fast-cycling course increases. This phase also includes the treatment of residual depressive or dysthymic symptoms, the control of affective instability, as well as pre relapse and early relapse disorders, including their rapid detection and timely intensification of thymoanaleptic therapy.

3) *Prophylactic therapy* is aimed at preventing the development of new episodes of the disease phase. For unipolar depression, small doses of serotonergic antidepressants or carbamazepine (finglepsin, tegretol) are usually used; for bipolar, lithium salts, carbamazepine or valproic acid salts (Depakine, etc.) are used. Prophylactic therapy may be given indefinitely, but not less than 1 year, so that its effectiveness can be evaluated. If there is a history of more than two recurrent depressive episodes, prophylactic therapy is necessary.

Before starting treatment, the patient should always be informed that depression is a medical condition and not a manifestation of fatigue or weakness of character, so it is necessary to observe the medication regimen. It should be explained that the drugs show their effect after 4-6 weeks, they are not addictive, although unpleasant feelings are possible in case of abrupt withdrawal of treatment. Prophylactic therapy in 70-80% of patients avoids the risk of relapse. Patients and relatives of patients should be informed about the first manifestations of depression, at the appearance of which they should immediately consult a physician [1, 62, 64].

5. Analysis of the clinical structure of anxiety-depressive disorders in outpatient practice and innovative approaches to their therapy

The world psychiatric practice has a rich experience in the organization of psychiatric care in primary health care. At the present stage of development of psychiatric service in the Republic of Kazakhstan a new concept of interaction of specialized psychiatric institutions with primary health care institutions was developed, which is reflected in the Order of the Ministry of Health of the RK №13404 of March 5, 2016. "On approval of the Standard of organizaticn of medical and social care in the field of mental health to the population of the Republic of Kazakhstan". [9,10]. According to the provisions of Chapter 2, item 2 of the given order, the competence of medical personnel of primary health care includes prescription of treatment, at establishment of diagnoses of boundary mental and behavioral disorders among which affective (anxious-depressive) disorders occupy the leading place: F32.0 "Depressive light episode"; F43.2 "Adaptation disorder"; F41.2 "Mixed anxious-depressive disorder"; F45 "Somatoform disorder"; F06.6
"Organic emotionally labile (asthenic) disorder"; F54
"Psychological and behavioral factors associated with disorders or diseases classified under other headings" (psychosomatic disorders). Social and economic importance of the problem of anxiety-depressive disorders, the urgency of which is reflected in the priority directions of healthcare development in the Republic of Kazakhstan, causes the necessity to study and introduce modern methods of their diagnostics and treatment into the general clinical practice.

In order to develop effective diagnostic and treatment methods for anxiety-depressive disorders with sleep disorders in general clinical practice, we analyzed the observation and therapy of 50 patients with anxiety-depressive disorders who received treatment in outpatient settings in Nur-Sultan and Almaty (2019-2020).

Distribution of examined patients by sex and age is shown in Table 1 and Figure 1

Table 1 Distribution of surveyed patients by sex and age

Age	Women		Men		T ot al :	
	A .c h.	%	A .c h.	%	A .c h.	%
21-30 years old	4	10, 5	6	50	1 0	2 0
31-40 years old	1 8	47, 4	2	16,7	2 2	4 4
41-50 years	1 0	26, 3	2	16,7	1 1	2 2
51-60 years old.	4	10, 5	2	16,6	5	1 0
61 years of age and older	2	5,2	-	-	2	4
Total:	3 8	10 0	1 2	100	5 0	1 0 0 0

A.h. - absolute number

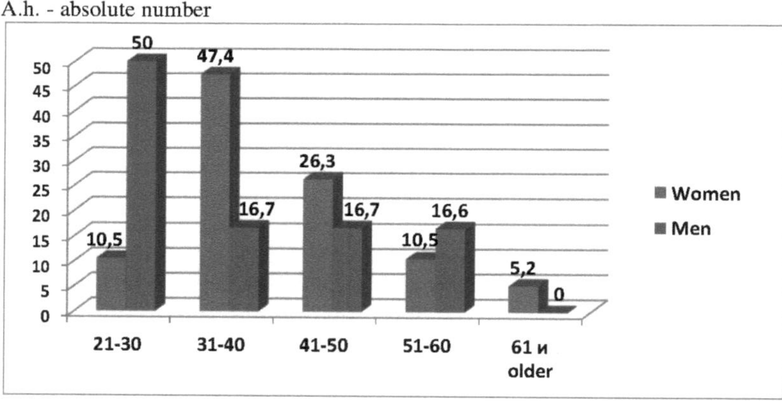

Figure 1 - Distribution of surveyed patients with anxiety-depressive disorders by gender and age group (%).

The data presented in Table 1 and Figure 1 show that the majority of those examined were women - 76%, the proportion of men was more than three times less - 24%. Patients aged 31-40 years prevailed among women (47.4%), and patients at a relatively younger age, 21-30 years (50%), prevailed among men. Thus, the data obtained in the study allow us to conclude that among patients with anxiety-depressive disorders receiving treatment in outpatient settings, persons of young working age from 21 to 50 years (86%) prevail, which determines the relevance of timely antidepressive therapy for these patients, starting from the PHC level.

The study of the medical history of the examined patients showed that in most cases, acute and prolonged psychotraumatic situations prevailed among the factors that could be attributed to the causes of the anxiety-depressive disorder - psychogenic anxiety-depressive disorders accounted for 60%.

The anxiety-depressive disorders were of somatogenic nature much less frequently - 34% - these disorders occurred in direct connection with an objective somatic disease and were in essence a reaction to the disease. In a few cases, the etiopathogenesis of the anxiety-depressive disorders revealed in the examined patients was dominated by exogenous-organic factors - 6%, as shown in Figure 2.

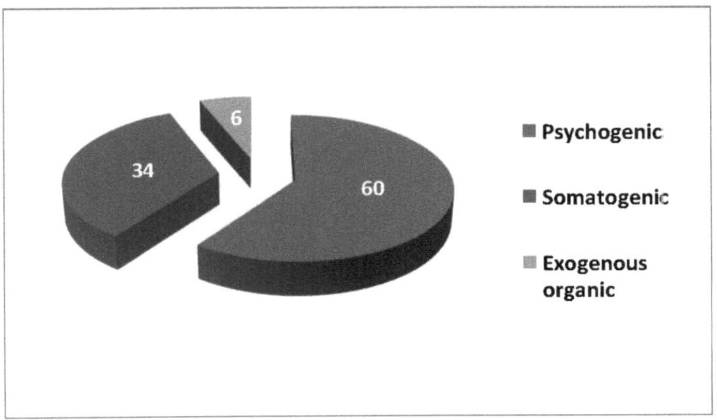

Figure 2 - Distribution of those examined according to the leading etiopathogenetic factor of anxiety-depressive disorders (%).

The data presented in Table 2 and Figure 3 suggest that younger individuals aged 21 to 40 years (80%) prevailed among patients with psychogenic depression, whereas middle-aged individuals aged 31 to 50 years (88.2%) prevailed among patients with somatogenic depression.

Table 2 Etiopathogenetic factors of anxiety-depressive disorders in selected age groups of patients examined

Genesis-depressive disorders	Age groups						%
	21-30 years	31-40 years	41-50 years	51-60 years	61 years old and older	Total:	
Psychogenic	9	15	3	3	-	30	60
Somatogenic	-	7	8	1	1	17	34
Exogenous organic	1	-	-	1	1	3	6
Total:	10	22	11	5	2	50	100
%	20	44	22	10	4	100	

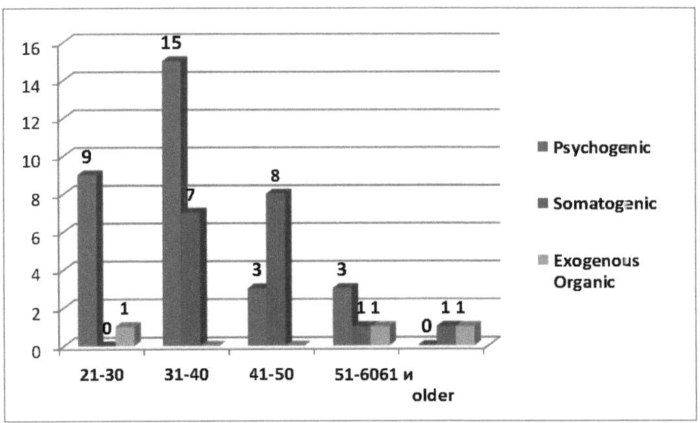

Figure 3 Etiopathogenesis of depressive-anxiety disorders in selected age groups (in absolute numbers).

Patients with anxiety-depressive disorders under observation were treated according to the updated Protocols for the Diagnosis and Treatment of Mental and Behavioral Disorders:

"Depression without Psychotic Symptoms" and "Neurotic Disorders" with the use of the modern antidepressant Mianserin (Menser), the choice of which was justified by the results of international studies, testifying from the position of evidence-based medicine about its effectiveness, safety and good tolerability in the treatment of anxiety-depressive disorders with sleep disturbances.

Mianserin (Menser) is a modern tetracycline antidepressant of the latest generation, with minimal risk of side effects and drug interactions, and thus is the drug of choice in treating patients with depressive disorders in the clinic of various mental disorders, in connection with which Mianserin is included in the British National Formulary [66] and in the Kazakh National Formulary.

The uniqueness of the antidepressant Mianserin is its high efficacy, comparable in strength of thymoanaleptics with amitriptyline, combined with additional positive effects - sleeping pills and anti-anxiety. Mianserin has a number of advantages: unlike commonly used tricyclic antidepressants: it is better tolerated and in therapeutic doses does not affect the cardiovascular system, does not cause anticholinergic effects, and does not affect dopaminergic conduction [67,68].

Due to the low risk of drug interactions, Mianserin combines well with neuroleptics and other antidepressants, particularly serotonin reuptake inhibitors [69], as well as medications used to treat concomitant somatic pathology. According to international studies, the use of Mianserin has proven to be most effective in anxiety-depressive disorders, including in patients with severe agitation, anxiety, and sleep disturbances [70,71]. According to recent scientific data, Mianserin is one of the most commonly used antidepressants in Europe for the treatment of sleep disorders in patients with various psychiatric disorders

[72].

Administration of Mianserin has a favorable effect on the recovery of sexual function impaired by other psychotropic medications. Mianserine has greater activity at adrenergic receptors than Mirtazapine and a more pronounced anti-anxiety effect (73). Mianserine, as a drug with few side effects, is widely used in Europe, especially in elderly patients, and it improves sleep and reduces anxiety from the first days of use, which is beneficial for the creation of compliance conditions (74).

Patients were followed up for 3 months, with follow-up examinations by physicians once every 2 weeks. Mianserin (Menser) was administered to patients at 30 mg. per day once at night.

The effectiveness of applied therapy was ***monitored*** by the dynamics of reduction of depressive and anxiety disorders with registration of indicators of anxiety and depression levels on psychometric scales.

Safety control was performed by active detection of adverse events during the use of Mianserin (Menser) according to the Instructions for Medical Use of this medicine, as well as by additional registration of all arising adverse events within the study period. Tolerability assessment and recording of side effects was performed using the Side Effect Rating Scail (UKU).

Results of clinical observations.

The baseline clinical level of depression and anxiety in the examined patients was determined at the first visit to the doctor using psychometric scales (HADS, HDRS, and HAM-A). Depressive disorders of borderline level were predominantly of mild to moderate severity. Depression severity scores on the Hamilton Depression Rating Scale (HDRS-17) ranged from 8 to 19, with an average of 12.3, corresponding to qualification of the condition as depressive disorder of average severity. The distribution of patients according to the severity of depression depending on the etiology is shown in Table 3.

Table 3 Distribution of patients by baseline severity of depression depending on etiological factors

Etiological factors	Baseline level of depression severity			
	Light	**Medium**	**Heavy**	**Average HDRS-17 score**
Psychogenic	15	15	-	13,2
Somatogenic	8	7	2	**15,8**
Exogenous Organic	1	2	-	8,0
Total:	**24 (48%)**	**24 (48%)**	**2 (4%)**	**12,3**

The data presented in Table 3 show that when assessing the depth of depression on the psychometric HDRS-17 scale, the severity of depressive disorders in the clinic of somatogenic depression was slightly higher than in psychogenic and exogenic-organic depressive disorders. Overall, mild depressive disorders and moderate depression were detected in equal numbers (48% each) among the examined patients, as shown in Figure 4.

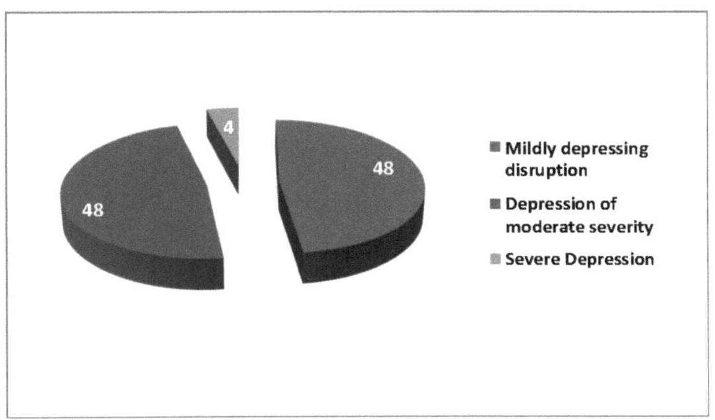

Figure 4 - Distribution of the cohort of examinees according to the severity of the initial level of depressive disorders (%).

The baseline level of anxiety was assessed using the HAM-A psychometric scale. According to the data obtained, the level of anxiety in the examined patients ranged from 11 to 27 points with a clear predominance of patients with an average level of anxiety, the average score for the general population of patients being 15.7. It should be noted that the highest mean level of anxiety (18.3 points) was detected in patients with psychogenic anxiety-depressive disorders, as shown in Table 4 and Figure 5.

Table 4 Distribution of patients according to the severity of the initial level of anxiety depending on etiological factors

Etiological factors	Initial level of severity of anxiety			
	Light	Medi um	Heavy	Average NAM-A score
Psychogenic	8	15	7	**18,3**
Somatogenic	6	8	3	18,0
Exogenous Organic	1	2	-	11.0
Total:	**15 (30%)**	**25 (50%)**	**10 (20%)**	**15,7**

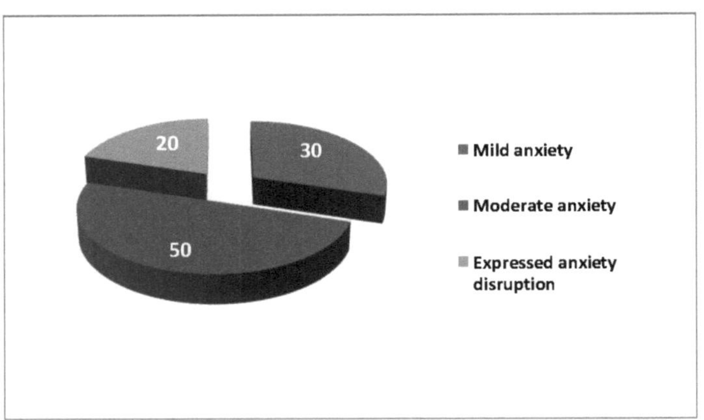

Figure 5 - Distribution of the population of patients examined according to the severity of the initial level of anxiety (%).

Thus, an objective assessment of the initial level of clinical condition of the examined patients showed that individuals with mild to moderate depression, which was accompanied by anxiety disorders of mostly moderate severity, predominated among the study subjects. The small number of patients with major depressive disorder (2 cases) can be explained by the outpatient care, since usually such patients are referred to a hospital for treatment. The fact of greater depth of depressive symptoms in somatogenic depressions and higher anxiety scores in psychogenic depressions is noteworthy.

Dynamics of depressive disorders during therapy with Mianserin (Menser) during 3 months of observation with registration of Depression Depression Scale score

Hamilton's HDRS-17 during patients' bi-weekly visits (Table 5 and Figures 6 and 7).

Table   Dynamics of the HDRS-17 Depression Depression Severity Scale during therapy with Mianserin (Menser) within 3 months

Etiopathogenesis of depressive disorder	Doctor's visits					
	1-й	2-й	3-й	4-й	5-й	6-й
Psychogenic	13.2	11.1	9.1	8.4	6.4	6.5
Somatogenic	15.8	14.7	13.1	10.7	8.3	6.7
Exogenous	8.0	8.0	7.0	7.0	1.0	1.0
Total (average score):	**12.3**	**11.6**	**9.7**	**8.7**	**5.4**	**4.7**

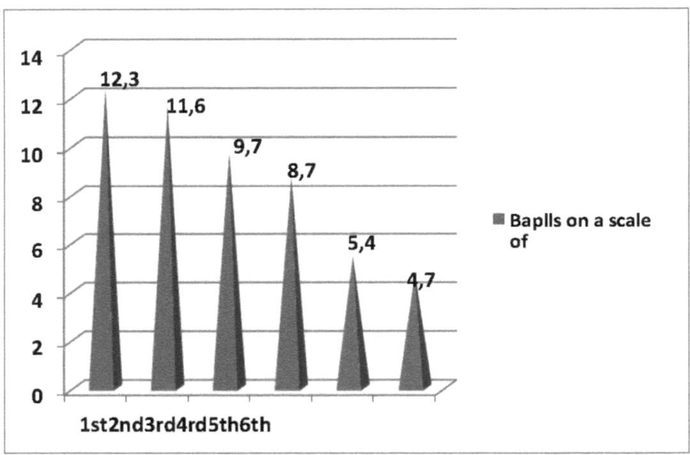

Figure 6 Dynamics of Depression Depression Depression Scale scores
ı HDRS-
17 during therapy with Mianserin (Menser) for 3 months (mean score).

The data presented in Table 5 and Figure 6 demonstrate convincingly the positive dynamics in the clinic of depression on the background of therapy with Mianserin (Menser) at a dose of 30 mg at night: while the mean HDRS-17 baseline depression score was 12.8, approaching the qualification of the condition as "depressive disorder of medium severity," after two weeks of therapy this score was reduced to 11.6, which would qualify as "mild depressive disorder. By week 8, the HDRS-17 score decreased to 5.4, indicating an absence of depressive disorder. Thus, in the course of clinical observations, objective data were obtained, indicating that during outpatient treatment of mild to moderate depression with Mianserin (Menser), a fairly pronounced positive dynamics in the reduction of depressive symptoms was observed by the end of the second week of treatment. By the end of the second month of taking this drug (8 weeks), most patients had no symptoms of depression, and it was possible to continue supportive treatment according to international standards for up to 6 months.

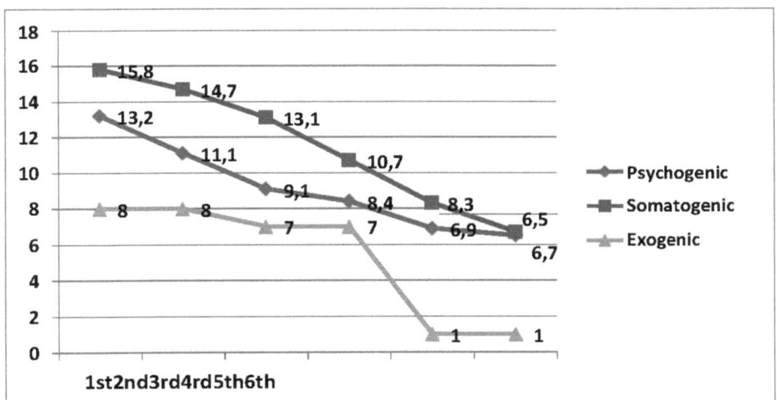

Figure 7 Dynamics of Depression Depression Depression Scale HDRS-17 during therapy with Mianserin (Menser) for 3 months in patients with different genesis of depressive disorder.

The data demonstrated in Figure 7 show that regardless of the genesis of the depressive disorder, the use of Mianserin (Menser) showed a positive trend in the reduction of depressive symptoms on the HDRS-17 scale. Notably, despite a higher HDRS-17 score in patients with somatogenic vs. psychogenic depressions, by the patient's 6th visit to the physician, treatment was successful in both the former and the latter, with the more severe somatogenic depression being more effectively reduced than the psychogenic one. Over the same period of therapy, somatogenic depressive disorders were reduced by 58.8% and psychogenic by 49.2%. Exogenous-organic depressions, although mild in severity at the initial examination, also had positive dynamics until the depressive disorders almost completely disappeared.

The *dynamics of anxiety disorders during therapy with Mianserin (Menser) during* 3 months of follow-up with recording of Hamilton Anxiety Scale (HAM-A) anxiety scores during patient visits every two weeks (Table 6 and Figures 8 and 9).

Table 6 Dynamics of NAM-A anxiety scores during therapy with Mianserin (Menser)

within 3 months

Etiopathogenesis of anxiety-depressive disorder	Doctor's visits					
	1-й	2-й	3-й	4-й	5-й	6-й
Psychogenic	18,3	16,1	13,4	11,2	8,5	6,1
Somatogenic	18,0	16,7	14,7	12,0	7,3	5,8
Exogenous	11,0	11,0	7.0	4,0	2,0	2,0
Total (average score):	15,7	14,6	11,7	9,1	5,9	4,6

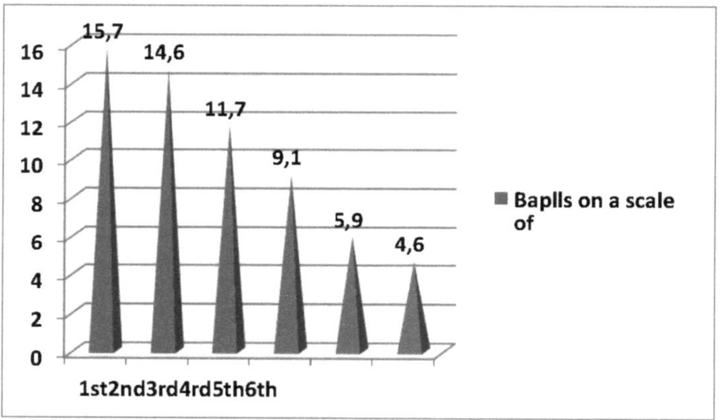

Fig. 8 NAM-A anxiety scores during therapy with Mianserin (Menser) over 3 months (mean score).

The data presented in Table 6 and Figure 8 demonstrate convincingly the positive dynamics of anxiety disorders against the background of therapy with Mianserin (Menser) at a dose of 30 mg at night: while the mean baseline NAM-A anxiety score was 15.7, which corresponded to "moderate anxiety disorder," after two weeks of therapy this index decreased to 14.6, which allowed to qualify the patients as anxiety disorders of medium severity.
"mild anxiety disorder." By the 8th week of therapy, the NAM-A score decreased to 5.9, indicating the absence of signs of anxiety. Thus, in the course of clinical observation, the following results were obtained

objective data showing that the treatment of depressive states, the clinical picture of which reveals symptoms of anxiety, with Mianserin (Menser) in an outpatient setting by the end of the first week of treatment there is a fairly pronounced reduction of the anxiety component of depression, and after 6 weeks - a complete reduction of anxiety.

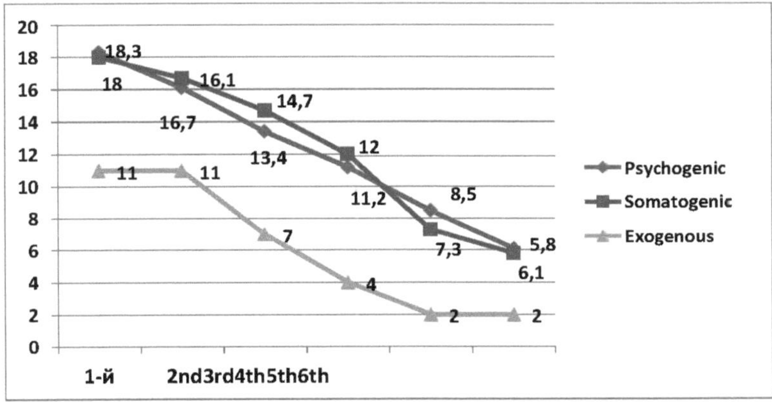

Figure 9 Dynamics of NAM-A anxiety scores during therapy with Mianserin (Menser) for 3 months in patients with different genesis of depressive disorder.

The data demonstrated in Figure 9 indicate that anxiety levels in both psychogenic and somatogenic depressions were effectively reduced by therapy with Mianserin (Menser) with the same degree of anxiety reduction at the observation intervals corresponding to the visits to the doctor (after 2 weeks). The initial level of anxiety disorders in the exogenous organic depression clinic was significantly lower, could initially be qualified as "mild anxiety," which also underwent rapid reduction. This allows us to conclude that therapy with the antidepressant Mianserin (Menser) effectively relieves anxiety symptoms in the clinic of depression regardless of their genesis. On the whole, the anxiety index in the examined patients decreased by 70% during the period of observation.

When comparing the rate of reduction of depressive disorders and reduction of anxiety severity on the background of therapy with Mianserin (Menser), it can be noted that during the month of treatment, depression scores decreased by 21.8% and anxiety by 25.5%. This allows us to conclude that the anti-anxiety effect of Mianserin (Menser) is ahead of its antidepressant effect. This has significant value IN terms of   selecting a combination therapy   for anxiety-depressive disorders. It is well   known that   almost   all   modern antidepressants (SSRIs and others) start to show their antidepressant (thymoanaleptic) effect only by the end of the first and sometimes second week of therapy, and in order to relieve anxiety at first it is recommended to add a tranquilizer to these drugs (especially if the antidepressant has stimulating effect). The present analysis of clinical observations of therapy of anxiety-depressive disorders with the antidepressant Mianserin (Menser) showed its good and early effectiveness in relieving anxiety disorders, which allows its use as monotherapy, and, therefore, gives an opportunity to reduce the cost of treatment.

Sleep disturbances in patients with anxiety-depressive disorders and their correction during therapy with Mianserin (Menser)

The symptom complex of a depressive episode (according to ICD-10) includes not only hypothymia, anhedonia and decreased activity, fatigue and decreased self-esteem, but also sleep disorders: presomnic, intrasomnic and postsomnic disorders.

During observation of patients with anxiety-depressive disorders, we used the International Diagnostic Criteria for Sleep Disorders (2005):

The presence of three or more of the following 7 signs continuously (more than one month) or intermittently (more than three months):

It takes more than 30 minutes to fall asleep;

-all night long, thoughts are going through my head;

-fear of not being able to sleep;

-frequent awakenings during the night;

-early awakenings and inability to go back to sleep;

-depressed mood and depression;

-unmotivated anxiety, fear.

Types of sleep disorders depending on the etiology of anxiety-depressive disorders in the examined patients are presented in Table 7 and Figures 10, 11.

Table 7 Types of sleep disorders depending on the etiology of anxiety-depressive disorders

Sleep disturbances	Psychogenic	Somatogenic	Exogenous-organic	Total:

	A.ch.	%	A.ch.	%	A.ch.	% e	A.h...	%
Presumption	18	60	5	29,4	-	-	23	46
Intrasomnical	9	30	10	58,9	3	100	22	44
Post-somniac	3	10	2	11,7	-	-	5	10
Total:	30	100	17	100	3	100	50	100

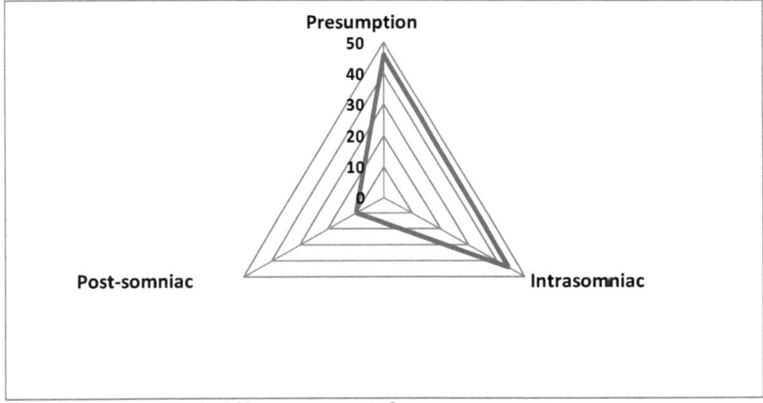

Figure 10-Ratio of different types of trespasses
of patients examined (%).

The data presented in Figure 10 show that almost all of the patients with anxiety-depressive disorders examined complained of sleep disorders at the initial examination. Most frequently, patients complained of difficulty falling asleep and frequent awakenings in the middle of the night with anxiety attacks. According to the findings:

Presomnic disorders (46%). The most frequent complaints of patients were difficulty falling asleep. Many patients noted
"rituals of going to bed," as well as "fear of bed" and fear of "not going to sleep.

Intrasomniac disorders (44%) included complaints of frequent nocturnal awakenings, after which patients could not fall asleep for a long time, and feelings of "superficial", "shallow" sleep.

Post-somnic disorders (10%) were observed less frequently, occurring in the immediate period after awakening. Patients complained about the problem of early morning awakening, decreased capacity for work, and "brokenness.

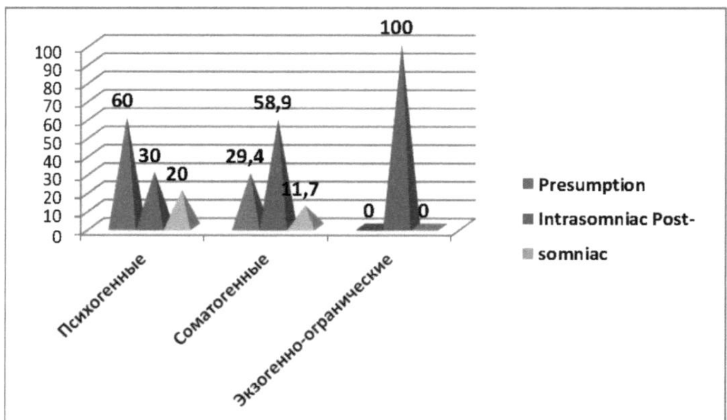

Figure 11 Comparative Characteristics of Individual Types of Violations sleep depending on the etiopathogenesis of anxiety-depressive disorders (%)

The data presented in Figure 11 show that presomnic disorders predominated in patients with psychogenic anxiety-depressive disorders (60%). These patients associated sleep disorders with the psychotraumatic situations they were experiencing. They said that they lay in bed for a long time thinking over disturbing facts, looking for a way out of the conflict. Often the psychologically traumatic situation was replayed in nightmares.

Patients with somatogenic anxiety-depressive disorders had intrasomnic disorders more frequently (58.9%). Waking up in the middle of the night was often associated with fears about their somatic health, listening to the heart, getting out of bed to check blood pressure, temperature, etc., then there was anxiety about the impossibility of falling asleep again, which kept them from falling asleep again.

In patients with the exogenous-organic nature of anxiety-depressive disorders (there were only 3 such patients), intrasomniac disorders also predominated.

Dynamics of sleep disorders in patients with anxiety-depressive disorders against the background of therapy with Mianserin (Menser).

The dynamics of sleep disorders in the course of the study were monitored by patients' subjective evaluation of sleep quality and recorded during the visits with appropriate scores:

10 points - sleep disturbances are pronounced and persistent

7 points - sleep disturbances are moderately pronounced, persistent

5 points - sleep disorders are moderately pronounced,

episodic 3 points - mild sleep disorders
0 points - normal sleep

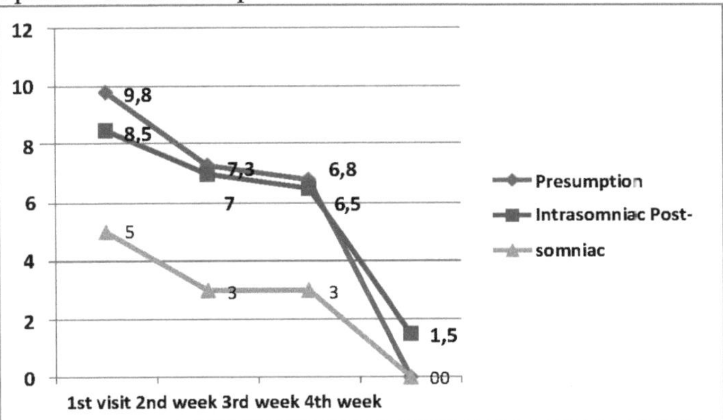

Figure 12 - Dynamics of individual types of sleep disorders in patients with anxiolytic-depressive disorders during therapy with Mianserin (Menser).

The data presented in Figure 12 show that positive dynamics was observed in patients with anxiety-depressive disorders against the background of Menser therapy at a dose of 30 mg at night. The most frequently observed presomnic disorders were characterized by patients as distressing and persistent in most cases. Often these patients had already been taking various drugs to improve sleep (somnol, phenazepam, dimedrol, various herbs, etc.) before starting this therapy without a persistent positive effect. Upon prescription of Menser, the patients noted improvement in falling asleep literally from the first days of therapy, and by the end of the 1st month of taking this drug, the patients managed to normalize their sleep if they observed the sleep regime (tried to fall asleep at the same time every day). Similar positive dynamics were observed for other types of sleep disorders (intrasomniac and postsomniac), but Menser's fast action and efficacy were more pronounced for presomniac disorders. Thus, in the course of this study, we managed to establish that of all clinical effects of Mianserin (Menser) the earliest is its favorable effect on sleep normalization, the anti-anxiety effect is manifested within the 1st week, and the actual antidepressant effect in most cases began to manifest from the 2nd week of this drug administration.

Security Control:

During this study, only one patient experienced an undesirable side effect of Mianserin (Menser), which was manifested by allergic

reactions with facial edema. After discontinuation of the drug, these phenomena rapidly reduced and did not require additional therapeutic measures. No other undesirable side effects of Mianserin (Menser) were observed in the examined patients. This demonstrates its good tolerability and safety and allows recommending Mianserin (Menser) for wide use in the treatment of anxiety-depressive disorders in outpatient settings, including general medical practice.

Discussion of the results of the study and conclusions

As a result of the carried out research the new data about sex and age peculiarities of disorders of anxious-depressive spectrum among outpatients in some regions of the Republic of Kazakhstan (Nur-Sultan, Almaty) were obtained. Peculiarities of clinic and course of depressive disorders in the structure of mental and behavioral disorders of borderline level were studied. Modern methods of revealing and diagnostics of anxious-depressive disorders with the use of international psychometric scales as well as effective methods of treatment of depressive and neurotic disorders with the use of modern antidepressants were adapted and introduced into the out-patient clinical practice. Data were obtained on the efficacy and safety of the use of Mianserin (Menser) for the treatment of anxiety-depressive disorders with sleep disorders in outpatient settings.

Conclusions:

1. Among patients with anxiety-depressive disorders requiring antidepressant therapy in outpatient settings, the predominant age group is young, of working age from 21 to 50 years (83.3%).

2. In the majority of cases among the factors which could be attributed to the reasons of occurrence of the anxious-depressive disorder, acute and prolonged psychotraumatic situations prevailed - psychogenic anxious-depressive disorders made up 60%. Considerably less frequently anxious-depressive disorders had somatogenic character - 34 % - these disorders have arisen in direct connection with objectively occurring somatic disease and in essence were a reaction to illness. In a few cases, exogenous-organic factors dominated in the etiopathogenesis of the anxiety-depressive disorders found in the examined patients - 6%.

Among patients with psychogenic depression, younger individuals between 21 and 40 years of age prevailed (80%), whereas among patients with somatogenic depression, middle-aged individuals between 31 and 50 years of age prevailed (88.2%).

3. An assessment of the baseline level of depressive disorders in the examined patients showed that mild depression and moderate depression severity were detected in equal numbers (48% each). The small number of patients with major depressive disorder (2 cases) can be explained by the outpatient care, since usually such patients are referred to a hospital for treatment. The fact of greater depth of depressive symptoms in somatogenic depressions and higher anxiety scores in psychogenic depressions is noteworthy.

4. In the process of clinical observation, objective data were obtained

showing that during treatment of mild to moderate depression with Mianserin (Menser) in outpatient settings, by the end of the second week of treatment, there was a fairly pronounced positive trend in the reduction of depression symptoms. By the end of the second month of taking this drug (8 weeks), most patients had no symptoms of depression, and it was possible to continue supportive treatment according to international standards for up to 6 months.

5.   With the use of Mianserin (Menser), there was a positive dynamics of depression symptom reduction on the HDRS-17 scale regardless of the genesis of the depressive disorder. Moreover, despite the higher HDRS-17 score in patients with somatogenic vs. psychogenic depressions, by the 6th visit of the patient to the doctor, treatment was successful both in the first and in the second case: the more severe depression of somatogenic nature was reduced more effectively (a 58.8% reduction) vs. psychogenic depression (49.2%).

6. In the process of clinical observation, objective data were obtained showing that during therapy with Mianserin (Menser) in outpatient conditions of depressive states, the clinical picture of which reveals symptoms of anxiety, a fairly pronounced reduction in the anxious component of depression was observed by the end of the first week of treatment, and after 6 weeks - a complete reduction of anxiety.

7. Therapy with the antidepressant Mianserin (Menser) effectively relieved anxiety symptoms in the clinic of depression regardless of their genesis. Anxiety levels in both psychogenic and somatogenic depressions effectively decreased with the same degree of anxiety reduction during the observation intervals corresponding to the visits to the doctor. Overall, the anxiety severity index in the examined patients decreased by 70% during the observation period.

8.   The present analysis of clinical observations of therapy of anxiety-depressive disorders with the antidepressant Mianserin (Menser) showed that its anti-anxiety effect is superior to its antidepressant effect. This allows its use as monotherapy, and, consequently, makes it possible to reduce the cost of treatment.

9. Virtually all of the patients with anxiety-depressive disorders examined complained of abnormalities during their initial examination.

sleep. Presomniac disorders predominated in patients with psychogenic anxiety-depressive disorders (60%), and intrasomniac disorders predominated in patients with somatogenic and exogenous-organic anxiety-depressive disorders (58.9%).

10. Against the background of therapy with Menser at a dose of 30 mg. at night, a positive dynamics was traced in patients with anxiety and depressive disorders with respect to sleep disorders. The rapidity of action and efficacy of Mianserin (Menser) was more pronounced with respect to presomnic disorders.

11. During the present study, we were able to establish that of all the clinical effects of Mianserin (Menser), the earliest is its favorable effect on sleep normalization, the anti-anxiety effect is manifested during the 1st week,

and the actual antidepressant effect in most cases began to appear from the 2nd week of this medication.

12. The results of this study showed that when using the antidepressant Mianserin (Menser) in outpatient settings, undesirable side effects are extremely rare (a single case of allergic reaction), it is well tolerated by patients and can be recommended for wide use in the treatment of anxiety-depressive disorders in general medical practice.

6. Clinical observations and their analysis

Patient I., 48 years old.

Heredity: my father was a stiff, directive, died at the age of 57 from a heart attack, my mother was anxious, mistrustful.

Past medical history: only child in the family, parents divorced when the girl was 6 years old. She grew up and developed according to her age, together with the general education, attended art school. After school she went to the university, entered the Faculty of Economics, but did not work in her field of study, due to childcare. Subsequently, she assisted her husband in business. She is married and has a grown-up daughter. She characterizes her relationship with her husband as conflictual and tense. Husband abuses alcohol, periodically had parallel relations, of which the patient became aware, however marriage was preserved due to "common business and common home". Altered mental condition within the last 3 years, when she first sought psychiatric help, due to disturbed night sleep, loss of appetite, decreased background mood, irritability, decreased productivity at work, anxiety, episodes of panic states accompanied by rise in arterial pressure, feeling of shortness of breath, increased pulse rate. The condition was qualified as

"Mixed anxiety-depressive disorder (F41.2). She was treated as an outpatient and was recommended to take atarax (50 mg per day) and duloxetine (60 mg per day). Slightly improved during treatment, but discontinued on her own two weeks later due to nausea, which   she felt was the result of   the   drugs. She was   convinced that

"will pull herself together and cope by herself. However, against the background of the absence of therapy, her condition worsened again after 3 months, which was the basis for a second visit to a specialist. Depression of mood with anxious-apathic accent, constant insomnia, painful sensations of various localizations ("heart compression", back pain, headaches) dominated the clinical picture of disease. Panic attacks became more pronounced and frequent and occurred both spontaneously and after regular conflicts in the family. At that time his therapeutic program included phenazepam (1 mg per day), amitriptyline (75 mg per day), psychotherapeutic correction in the form of rational psychotherapy. Against the background of amitriptyline, the patient's tachycardia increased, which was the reason for changing the drug to mirtazapine (myrtel - 30 mg per day). Against the background of this scheme of treatment and psychotherapeutic work, positive dynamics was noted in the condition, but due to weight gain, the patient discontinued treatment on her own. However, somatic symptoms persisted and the patient continued to be examined by internists (neurologist, cardiologist, gastroenterologist, endocrinologist). No significant pathology was detected. Another worsening of her condition was characterized by increased internal tension, painful sensations in the head, neck and spine, painful sensations in the abdomen, periods of increased BP, increased heart rate, (mostly after conflict situations). According to patient's words, divorce process, initiated by patient, contributed to worsening of her condition. When she sought help, she was in a depressed mood, occurring primarily in the first half of the day, insomnia, pronounced emotional lability (tearfulness). "I am completely disintegrated, everything hurts, I have lost the ability to enjoy life." On objective examination, the depressed mood background, injection of the sclerae (an objective sign of insomnia) drew attention. The patient noted that she had difficulty falling asleep, frequent nocturnal awakenings, lack of rest and vigor after a night's sleep. The patient's mental condition was classified as "Adaptation disorder. Mixed anxiety and depressive reactions. F43.22.». Treatment program included administration of mianserine (Menser), with initial dosage of 15 mg per day, with subsequent increase of dosage to 30 mg per day, and gidazepam in daily dose of 100 mg, rational psychotherapy. Already from the first week of therapy, both positive dynamics and good tolerance of the drugs were noted in the condition. Gidazepam was prescribed

for 3 weeks, and was subsequently discontinued. Menser was continued for 3 months at a daily dose of 30 mg. The patient noted good tolerability and efficacy of Menser, which increased adherence to treatment. During treatment, somato-vegetative symptoms of anxiety were completely leveled, sleep, mood and productive activity were restored.

Follow-up: (after 8 months). Patient's condition remains stable, mood is even, no complaints of sleep disturbances. She has reconciled with her husband and continues to conduct her business productively. Has plans for the future.

Observation Analysis:

The patient's mental and physical development was age-appropriate. Having successfully graduated from school and university, she was engaged in raising her daughter and helping her husband in business. Her personal life was ambiguous; in the presence of material well-being, her husband abused alcohol and did not always remain faithful. The first application for psychiatric help at the age of 45 years was preceded by intensification of conflicts with her husband. The clinical picture included symptoms of anxiety and depression, which were somewhat alleviated by outpatient treatment. The turnaround for psychiatric help occurred 4 months after the initial treatment. The clinical picture was dominated by disorders of the affective spectrum: depressed mood, with anxious-apathic accent, persistent insomnia, painful sensations of various localizations. Panic attacks became more expressed and frequent and occurred both spontaneously and after regular conflicts in the family. Prescribed therapy, though somewhat alleviating the condition, did not lead to the desired result, including due to the individual reaction to psychopharmacological medications. At the next worsening of the condition, manifested by the dominance of sleep disorders, symptoms of anxiety and depression, mianserine (Menser) was prescribed, which showed both high therapeutic effectiveness and good individual tolerance of the drug, which made it possible to increase adherence to treatment and achieve a high level of compliance.

This clinical example demonstrates quite convincingly the effectiveness of mianserine (Menser) for anxiety depression developing as part of an adjustment disorder.

Observation 2

Patient A., 38 years old.

Heredity: no father's data, parents divorced before the birth of the girl. The mother is calm and balanced in character.

Past medical history: only child in the family, raised by her mother and grandmother, with whom she was very close. Her early development was without any peculiarities, in her childhood she was engaged in singing and rhythmic gymnastics. After leaving school she went to the Department of Journalism, graduated successfully, but after graduation could not find the job she wanted ("I wanted to work in television, but there were no vacancies"), and decided to go to the Faculty of Law, "to follow in the footsteps of her mother, a successful lawyer. She is currently working as a lawyer. At the age of 28 she got married, has a 9-year-old son. Relationships in the marriage did not work out, "did not meet the characters", tried to build a new relationship, but also experienced a number of disappointments in the partners. At present she is raising a child on her own, noting that her husband has almost no involvement in supporting the child.

"it's all on me." Deterioration of the mental condition within the last 8 months, the change of a condition was preceded by a number of psychogenic events. She noted that her grandmother died a year and a half ago and felt the loss acutely, but "managed to pull herself together, did not show others the pain of loss. During the same period of time there were problems at work, which affected her financial situation. She was forced to change jobs. A year ago she met a young man, tried to build a relationship, but after a few months of a close relationship, was disappointed in her partner. She complained about sleep disorders - "I can't sleep", says that the process of falling asleep lasts for 2-3 hours, is accompanied by disturbing thoughts, images and memories, sleep is characterize   d by superficiality,   frequent   waking up,   morning tiredness, lack of sleep. "brokenness." There were also complaints of a lowered mood, constant internal tension, irritability, weakness, decreased concentration, and increased fatigue. The consequences of the unsatisfactory psychological state were errors in the process of work, which secondary caused a decrease in self-confidence, maintaining a negative self-esteem.   The condition was qualified as "Adaptation disorder. Prolonged depressive reaction. Agriptyne syndrome." The type of affect was characterized as astheno-depressive. Treatment program included administering atarax in a dosage of 25 mg per day (12.5 mg in the morning and in the evening) and myanserin (Menser) in a dosage of 30 mg per day (1 tablet in the evening), rational psychotherapy. From the first days of treatment, there was good tolerance of this regimen, which helped to decrease internal tension and restore sleep. After the first week of taking the medication, the patient noted a significant decrease in internal tension and improvement of the mood background. Atarax was continued for 2 weeks, and treatment was continued with Menser - 30 mg in the evening afterwards. After 8 weeks from the start of treatment, the patient evaluated her mental state as comfortable, anxiety was completely leveled, mood background stabilized,   functional activity and productivity   at work restored.   To   consolidate   the positive , it was recommended to continue taking Menser for 3 more weeks in a dosage of 30 mg in the evening, and then for 2 more weeks in a dosage of 15 mg in the evening.

Catamnesis: (after 1.5 years). Mental condition remained stable, mood background even, successfully continues lawyer's career.

Observational analysis: The patient's mental and physical development was consistent with her age. Her studies and professional career were successful, but in her personal life there were disappointments and difficulties in building close relationships with men. Change of mental condition was preceded by a number of psychogenic moments: death of favourite grandmother, problems at work, disappointment in trying to build family relationships. At the moment of treatment, the clinical picture of the disease was dominated by sleep disorders, a lowering of the mood, anxiety, heightened fatigability, and a decrease in productivity at work. The therapeutic program, including mianserin (Menser) from the first days of admission showed high therapeutic efficacy and good individual tolerability, stability of the positive changes achieved.

This clinical example is quite convincing evidence of the effectiveness of mianserine (Menser) for asthenic depression, agrippnic syndrome, developing as part of an adaptation disorder.

Observation 3

Patient K., 34 years old

Heredity: The grandmother on the mother's side was repeatedly treated in a psychiatric clinic for emotional disorders (depression). An aunt on the mother's side also sought psychiatric help and was treated in a psychiatric hospital for "a nervous breakdown. The father is calm and well-balanced by character, and the mother is described as anxious and restless.

Anamnesis: early development without any peculiarities, the youngest of two children, in junior high school she was engaged in artistic gymnastics, in high school she attended drama club, did vocals, often performed at school festivals. After graduating from high school I entered the university, majoring in Foreign Languages, after which I got a job at a school as an English teacher. At school, in addition to her professional duties, she actively participated in extra-curricular activities. She has been married since 22 years old and has two children, aged 11 and 7. She describes herself as a very responsible and sympathetic person: "I can't refuse anyone, even at the expense of my own interests", "I'm used to doing everything perfectly". She characterizes her husband as a kind and thoughtful man, "the breadwinner of the family. Mental changes

conditions since 2017, when symptoms of tension in the neck area, head, respiratory disorders - "could not breathe in", increased BP, accompanied by a sense of panic first appeared. Sleep was disturbed, the period of falling asleep lengthened up to 1.5-2 hours, early morning awakening appeared. Change of mental condition was preceded by husband's leaving the family for a month,

with real threat of divorce. She blamed herself for "not creating conditions for her husband," "spending a lot of time at work," "neglecting the house, not enough time with the childre   n. The patient reports that she was at that time "I managed to pull myself together, but after my husband returned to the family, the symptoms described above began to increase. I applied for help to a psychotherapist, took phenazepam (1 mg per day, amitriptyline 50 mg per day) and felt some improvement of my condition. She came to the conviction, that she could not combine work and household duties and decided to quit her favorite job, saying with regret that she missed her job, but due to "health problems" she could not go back to school. She has not worked for the past year, but notes that her "health continues to deteriorate." Even with periodic anti-anxiety medications (Adaptol, phenazepam) he continues to feel inner tension, unpleasant sensations in the heart area (tachycardia, pressing sensations) radiating to the left scapula. The BP is measured several times during the day, with values varying from 105 and 75 mmHg to 130 and 85 mmHg. She also reports panic attacks accompanied by a rise in BP to 140 and 90 mmHg. She also reported panic states accompanied by BP rising to 140 and 90 mmHg, respiratory disorders and pronounced fear of death, episodes of "body tremors" and "leg cramps". I began to read medical literature interpreting my own symptoms as signs of severe disease. Repeatedly examined by cardiologist, neurologist, pulmonologist. No significant pathology was found, she took neuroprotective and vasodilator medications, B-group vitamins, but her condition did not improve, which was a reason for further examination with the purpose of
"to find the cause of the bodily disorder. At the moment of seeking help there was expressed anxiety, anxiety about health problems, the patient noted the presence of constant thoughts about "a possible disease that specialists did not notice", she described in detail unkempt body sensations, showed concern about the constant deterioration of her health - "I'm 34 years old, I feel so sick". Her clinical condition at the moment of treatment was characterized by impaired mood, sleep, appetite, volitional activity was focused on health problems. At the time of referral, the condition was qualified as "Other mixed anxiety disorder F41.3, hypochondriac syndrome". Treatment was conducted on an outpatient basis, the treatment program included prescription of myanserin (Menser) in the first week at a dose of 15 mg per day, and 30 mg per day thereafter. During the first week, administration of Menserin was combined with phenazepam (1 mg per day), and thereafter Menserin was administered as monotherapy. Medication

the treatment program was accompanied by psychotherapeutic work. Positive dynamics in the patient's condition should be noted from the beginning of the second week of therapy, manifested by decreased anxiety, improved sleep and appetite. On the fourth week of therapy, the patient reported a significant decrease in internal tension, disappearance of panic states, decreased intensity of anxious thoughts, cessation of constant BP control. By week 8, discomfort in the heart area was eliminated, blood pressure stabilized, productivity in housework restored. To consolidate the positive state, it was recommended to continue taking Menser for another 5 weeks at a dosage of 30 mg in the evening, and then the maintenance dosage of 15 mg in the evening for another three weeks.

Catamnesis: (after 1 year). Mental condition remained stable, mood background was even, somato-vegetative symptoms were absent.

Analysis of observation: There was information in the anamnesis about maternal anxiety-depressive disorders. Mental and physical development of the patient corresponded to her age. Characteristic features of the patient had both the features of increased responsibility and high impressionability and emotionality. The patient sacrificed a successful professional career "for the sake of the family," but giving up her work did not improve her mental condition, but rather contributed to the increase of her anxiety and depression symptoms, intensifying intrapersonal conflict. At the moment of seeking help, somato-vegetative disorders, sleep disorders, decreased background mood, internal tension dominated the clinical picture of the disease. Due to the fact that in the clinical picture of the disease there were signs not only of anxiety, but also elements of conversion disorders ("body tremor, leg cramps"), hypochondria, signs of somatoform disorders, the condition was qualified as "Other mixed anxiety disorder F41.3, hypochondria syndrome". The therapeutic program including mianserine (Menser) from the first days of treatment showed high therapeutic efficacy and good tolerability of the drug, stability of the achieved positive changes.

This clinical example demonstrates quite convincingly the effectiveness of mianserine (Menser) for disorders of the anxiety-depression spectrum.

Conclusion

The modern development of clinical psychiatry involves the integration of specialized psychiatric care into broader medical practice.Depressive and anxiety disorders are the most common forms of psychiatric pathology. The social and economic costs associated with these disorders are great, and are often underestimated due to under-treatment and under-treatment.   have demonstrated   that those   suffering from depressive disorders   Numerous studies have shown that people with depressive disorders are more likely to seek help from general practitioners or, in rare cases, psychiatrists, psychotherapists and medical psychologists. In this regard, the role of general practitioners in the timely detection and adequate treatment of depression, which complicates the course of somatic diseases, significantly reduce the quality of life and the level of social functioning of patients, is increasing. Anxiety serves as a biological warning system,
which is activated by danger. Despite the abundance of special studies, including those conducted in recent decades, the problem of anxiety in psychiatry has not lost its relevance. The unflagging interest of psychiatrists in

anxiety states is evidence of their clinical and social importance for the solution of the problems of mental health protection of the population. The study of anxiety states is becoming increasingly relevant due to the fact that they most fully reflect the organism's maladaptive response to the pathogenic influence of the environment.

The wide prevalence of anxiety disorders in the population, the propensity for a prolonged course, accompanied by a significant decrease in the ability to work and quality of life of such patients, cause the need to develop and implement in practice effective methods of their timely diagnosis and treatment.

Currently, the possibilities for therapy of depressive and anxiety disorders have significantly expanded due to the emergence of a large number of new antidepressants. International studies have proved the effectiveness of therapy of depressive disorders with Mianserin (Menser), which, having a complex of pharmacological effects (antidepressant, anti-anxiety, sleeping pills), provides a new clinical approach to therapy of anxiety-depressive disorders with sleep disturbances. Practical absence of side effects, good tolerability and safety allow to recommend Mianserin (Menser) for therapy of anxiety-depressive disorders in general clinical practice patients at primary care level.

Applications

Appendix 1

Clinical variants of masked depression.

"Masks" in the form of psychopathological disorders
- anxiety-phobic (generalized anxiety disorder, anxious doubts, panic attacks, agoraphobia)
- Obsessive-compulsive disorder
- hypochondriac
- neurasthenic

"Masks" in the form of biological rhythm disturbances
- insomnia
- Hypersomnia

"Masks" in the form of vegetative, somatized and endocrine disorders
- Vascular dystonia syndrome, dizziness
- functional disorders of internal organs (hyperventilation syndrome, cardioneurosis, irritable bowel syndrome)
- neurodermatitis, skin itching
- anorexia, bulimia
- impotence, menstrual disorders

"Masks" in the form of algias
- cephalgia
- Cardialgia
- abdominalgia
- neuralgia
- Spondyloalgia
- pseudorheumatic algias

"Masks" in the form of pathocharacterological disorders
- addiction disorders (dipsomania, substance abuse, drug addiction)
- antisocial behavior (impulsivity, conflict)
- Hysterical reactions (touchy-feely, tearfulness, tendency to dramatize the situation, taking on the role of the patient, the desire to draw attention to one's ailments)

Glossary

Agitation is anxious agitation with a need for incessant movement.

Alexithymia is the inability to recognize, express and describe one's own feelings and state of mind.

Anhedonia - the inability to feel pleasant, a sense of contentment.

Anxious states are a group of syndromes manifested by the prevalence of anxiety, fears and other affective disorders, as well as vegetative symptoms (palpitations, sweating, tremors, etc.).

Anorexia - absence of desire to eat in the presence of physiological need for food. Anorexia nervosa is a persistent refusal to eat with preserved appetite due to mental illness, accompanied by pathological eating behavior (artificial vomiting, taking laxatives)

Asthenia is a condition of increased fatigue with hypersensitivity to normally neutral stimuli, emotional and vegetative lability, and sleep disorders.

Generalized anxiety disorder - chronic (at least 6 months) pathological anxiety with a pronounced feeling of internal tension, anxiety, unstable fears of ordinary content, excessive concern about current problems, possible health problems with a variety of vegetative disorders and other manifestations of bodily discomfort.

Hyperesthesia is heightened sensitivity to stimuli affecting the sensory organs. Mental hyperesthesia is characterized by hypersensitivity to psychotraumatic influences and even to neutral events perceived as traumatic, heightened emotional excitability, vulnerability, and increased exhaustion.

Hypothymia is a stable decrease in mood accompanied by a decrease in the intensity of one's emotional life, motor and mental activity. It is more often observed in cyclothymia and borderline states.

Dysthymia is an ICD-10 diagnostic category - chronic (lasting at least 2 years) depression of the non-psychotic level, with minimally expressed symptoms (even in periods of exacerbation, not only delirium, hallucinatory, or stupor symptoms are absent, but also ideas of guilt, suicidal thoughts or attempts, expressed psychomotor inhibition or agitation, which are typical for major depression)

Comorbidity is the coexistence of two or more syndromes (trans syndromic) or diseases (transnosologic) in one

patient, pathogenetically related to each other or coinciding in time.

Compliance is a conscious collaboration between physician, patient and family members. Compliance is a "therapeutic tool" that ensures the patient's interest in the treatment process, which promotes the accurate implementation of the doctor's recommendations and allows an objective judgment of the therapy's effectiveness.

Obsessions (obsessive-compulsive syndrome) - psychopathological conditions with the prevalence of thoughts, doubts, memories, notions, fears, cravings, actions, irresistibly, despite awareness of their morbidity.

Obsessive-compulsive disorder is a psychopathological condition with the predominance of obsessive thoughts (obsessions) and actions (compulsions).

Obsessive-phobic disorder is a psychopathological condition with the prevalence of obsessions and phobias.

Panic attack is an attack of sudden anxiety with fear (death, loss of self-control) and massive vegetative manifestations arising both in connection with certain circumstances and without reason.

Raptus - frenzied excitement, suddenly interrupted by depressive lethargy or stupor and accompanied by vitriolic longing, confusion, suicidal attempts.

Somatogenias are psychopathological disorders arising in diseases of internal organs as a result of a direct effect of somatic harm on the CNS.

Somatoform disorders is a diagnostic category in the ICD-10 that includes psychopathological disorders similar to manifestations of somatic pathology, which are excluded only by focused examination.

A phobia is a compulsive fear, a type of neurotic disorder. Phobias can be both isolated and multiple and can be combined with other disorders from the circle of obsessions (for example, obsessive-compulsive). Hypochondriacal phobias are a type of obsessive compulsion, the content of which is fear for life.

Frustration is one of the forms of psychopathological stress arising in a situation of disappointment and manifested by anger, irritation, guilt. Frustration causes insurmountable (or subjectively so perceived) difficulties.

Hospital Anxiety and Depression Scale (HADS)

Part I (assessment of the level of TRANSMISSION)
I feel tension, I feel uncomfortable 3 -
all the time
2 - often
1 - from time to time,
sometimes 0 - do not
experience at all
I feel afraid, as if something terrible is about to happen.
3 - definitely it is, and the fear is very great
2 - yes, it is, but the fear is not very great
1 - Sometimes, but it doesn't bother
me 0 - I don't experience it at all
Restless thoughts swirl in my head 3 - all
the time
2 - most of the time
1 - from time to time and not so
often I can easily sit down and
relax
0 - definitely it is 1 -
probably it is
2 - only occasionally,
that's so 3 - can't do it
at all
I experience internal tension or shudder 0 - not
at all
1 - sometimes
2 - often
3 - very often
I experience restlessness, I need to move all the time 3 - I
definitely do.
2 - I guess it is
1 - only to some extent, it's so 0 - I
don't experience at all
I get a sudden feeling of panic 3 - very
often
2 - more often than not
1 - not so often 0
- not at all

Part II (assessment of DEPRESSION)

What gave me great pleasure, and now gives me the same feeling.
0 - definitely it is 1 -
probably it is

2 - only to a very small extent, it is so
3 - it is not so at all
I am capable of laughing and seeing funny 0 in this or that event -
definitely it is
1 - I guess it is.
2 - only to a very small extent, it is so
0 - not at all capable of
I feel invigorated.
3 - I don't experience
it at all 2 - very rarely
1 - sometimes
0 - practically all the time
I feel like I started doing everything very slowly
3 - pretty much all the time
2 - often
1 - sometimes
0 - not at all
I'm not watching my
appearance 3 - definitely am
2 - I don't devote as much time to it as I need to 1 -
Maybe I've started to devote less time to it 0 - I'm
watching myself the same way I used to
I believe that my activities (activities, hobbies) can bring me a sense of
  satisfaction
0 - just as we usually do
1 - Yes, but not as much as before 2
- much less than usual 3 - I don't
think so at all
I can enjoy a good book   ,   a radio, and a good book.
or TV programs
0 - often
1 - sometimes
2 - seldom
3 - very rarely
Number of points:

0-7 points - Normal
8-10 points - subclinically expressed symptoms
More than 11 points - clinically expressed
symptoms

Hamilton Anxiety and Depression Scales

1. **Lowered mood** *(feelings of sadness, hopelessness, helplessness and inferiority)*

4 The patient expresses only these feelings both spontaneously and nonverbally.

3 Affective experiences are determined by non-verbal signs (facial expression, posture, nonverbal characteristics of the voice, crying or readiness to cry, etc.).

2 Spontaneously reports his or her experiences verbally (talks about them).

1 Reports his or her experiences only upon questioning.

0 Absent.

2. Guilt

4 Verbal hallucinations of an accusatory and judgmental nature and/or visual hallucinations of a threatening nature.

3 The present morbid condition is regarded as punishment; delusions of guilt.

2 Feelings and ideas of guilt or agonizing reflections on past mistakes (sins) and thoughts of punishment for those actions.

1 Ideas of self-abasement, self-deprecation; feels that he has let others down; feels that he is the cause of other people's suffering.

0 Absent.

3. Suicidal tendencies

4 Suicide attempt (any serious suicide attempt is scored 4 points).

3 Suicidal statements (thoughts) or gestures.

2 Desire for death or any thoughts about the possibility of your own death (ideas about not wanting to live)

1 Feeling that life is not worth living; expresses thoughts about the meaninglessness or low value of life.

0 Absent

4. Early insomnia (difficulty falling asleep)

2 Daily complaints about difficulty falling asleep.

1 Complaints of occasional difficulty falling asleep; it takes more than half an hour to fall asleep.

0 Absent.

5. Average insomnia

2 Multiple awakenings throughout the night (any rising out of bed during the night, with the exception of going to the toilet, is rated 2 points).

1 Complains of restless sleep (agitation and restlessness) throughout the night.

0 Absent.

6. Late insomnia (early awakenings)

2 Upon awakening, it is not possible to fall asleep again (final early awakening).

1 He wakes up early, but goes back to sleep.

0 Absent.

7. Work and activity (work and activity)

4 Refusal to work. Unable to work due to present illness. During an inpatient stay, the item is scored 4 if the patient does not show any activity other than the usual self-care activities or has difficulty even in this (cannot cope with routine household activities without assistance).

3 Significant decrease in activity and productivity. Decrease real time manifestation of activity or decreased productivity. In an inpatient unit, the item is scored 3 if the patient is engaged in any
activities (assistance to health care personnel, hobbies, etc.), other than normal self-care activities, for at least 3 hours a day.

2 Loss of interest in activity. Loss of interest in professional activities, work, and entertainment, determined directly by the patient's complaints or indirectly by the degree of indifference to
hesitation and hesitation (feeling that he has to force himself to work or do something; feeling the need to make an extra effort to be active).

1 Thoughts and feelings of inadequacy, feelings of fatigue and weakness related to activities (work or hobbies).

0 He has no difficulties

8. lethargy *(slowness of thinking and speech, impaired ability to concentrate, decreased motor activity)*

4 Total stupor

3 Expressed difficulties in interviewing

2 Noticeable (obvious) lethargy in conversation.

1 Mild (slight) lethargy in conversation.

0 Pace of thought and speech unchanged

9. Agitation (agitation)

4 He is constantly running his hands over and over, breaking his hands, biting his nails and lips, tearing his hair.

3 Mobility and restlessness

2 Restless movements of hands, hair rubbing ("play with hands, hair"), etc.

1 Anxiety.

0 Absent.

10. Mental Anxiety

4 Spontaneously expresses his or her anxious fears. Fear expressed without questioning.

3 Anxiety reflected in facial expression and speech.

2 Anxiety for insignificant reasons.

1 Subjective tension and irritability.

0 Absent.

11. **Anxiety somatic** *(physiological signs of anxiety: gastrointestinal - dry mouth,*

12. *Stomach pain, flatulence, diarrhea, dyspepsia, cramps, belching; cardiac*

vascular - palpitations, headaches; respiratory - hyperventilation, shortness of breath, shortness of breath; frequent urination, increased sweating)

4 Very severe, up to functional insufficiency (extremely severe).

3 Heavy (strong)

2 Medium

1 Weak

0 Not available

13. Gastrointestinal somatic disorders (symptoms)

Eating only with persistent compulsion. Needs.

2 prescription of laxatives and other medications that promote normal digestion.

1 Loss of appetite. Complains of lack of appetite, but eats independently without compulsion; has a feeling of heaviness in the stomach (stomach).

0 Absent.

14. Generalized symptoms

2 The distinct severity of any somatic symptom is given a score of 2.

1 Feeling of heaviness in limbs or back; back or head pain; muscle pain. Feeling of fatigue, loss of strength, or loss of energy.

0 Absent.

15. Sexual disorders
(genital symptoms) *(loss of libido, menstrual disorders)*

2 Clear expression of decreased libido (menstrual disorders)

1 Mild degree of decrease in libido. Mild severity of impairment.

0 Absent

16. Hypochondriacal disorders (hypochondria)

4 Hypochondriacal delusions (hypochondriacal delirium).

3 Frequent complaints, requests for help.

2 Particular (excessive) concern for one's health.

1 Increased interest in one's own body (self-absorption - one's own body).

0 Absent.

17. **Weight loss** *(evaluated by either item A or B)*

16 A. Assessment is made on the basis of anamnestic data

3 Significant weight loss, which is not estimable.

2 Apparent (according to the patient) weight loss. Loss of 3 or more kilograms.

1 Probable weight loss due to the present disease. Weight loss was 1 to 2.5 kg.

0 No weight loss was observed.

16 Б. The evaluation is made weekly according to the readings of the weights

3 It is not assessable.

2 Weight loss is more than 1 kg per week.

1 Weight loss is more than 0.5 kg per week.

0 Weight loss is less than 0.5 kg per week.

18. Attitude towards your illness (critical attitude towards the illness)

2 Complete lack of awareness of the disease. Does not consider himself sick.

1 Awareness of sickness; recognizes that he/she is sick, but attributes the causes of the illness to food, climate, overwork at work, viral infection, need for rest, etc.

0 Believes he/she is sick with depression. Awareness that he/she is sick with depression or some illness.

18. Diurnal fluctuations of the state. 18 A. Specify whether the condition worsens in the morning or in the evening

2 Deterioration in the evening.

Deterioration in the morning.

0 No change in composition (no diurnal fluctuations)

18 Б. If diurnal fluctuations in the condition are present, assess their severity

2 Expressed.

1 Weak.

0 The condition does not change (no diurnal fluctuations).

19. **Depersonalization and derealization** *(e.g., feeling that the world is unreal, nihilistic ideas)*

4 Completely cover the patient's consciousness (intolerable).

3 Strongly pronounced.

2 Moderately pronounced.

1 Weakly pronounced.

0 Absent.

20. Delusional disorders (paranoid symptoms)

3 Delusions of attitude and persecution.

2 Relationship Ideas.

1 Suspicion.

0 Absent.

21. Obsessive and compulsive disorders

2 Strongly pronounced (severe).

1 Weakly pronounced (mild).

0 Absent.

The total score is determined by the first 17 items (9 of which are scored from 0 to 4, and 8 from 0 to 2). The last four items of the Hamilton scale (items 18 through 21) are used to assess additional symptoms of depression and to determine subtypes of depressive disorder. Scores on these 4 items are not used in determining the severity of depression, and these scores are not considered in calculating the total Hamilton scale score, which determines the severity of depressive disorder.

The cumulative score of the first 17 points:

- 0-7 is normal
- 8-13 - mild depressive disorder
- 14-18 - depressive disorder of moderate severity
- 19-22 - severe depressive disorder
- more than 23 - depressive disorder of an extremely severe degree

List of references

1. Mosolov S. N. Clinical application of modern antidepressants. SPb. 1995. C. 564.
2. Wittchen H.U.. Report of the European College of Neuropsychopharmacology (ECMP) working group and the prevalence and burden of mental disorders in Europe (abstract). Bekhterev Review of Psychiatry and Medical Psychology 2005; 4:42 - 44.
3. Churkin A.A., Mikhailov V.I., Kasimova L.N. Mental health of the urban population. Moscow, Khabarovsk; 2000.
4. Ponizovsky A.M. Masked Depression // The Nurse and Midwife. - – M., 1988. - – №12. C. 36-40
5. Katona C., Livingston G. Comorbid depression in older people. (Lundbeck, DerRelief - Relieve Depression through Education) Martin Dunitz Ltd, London, 1997, 81p.
6. Cross-national comparisons of the prevalences and correlates of mental disorders // Bull. WHO. - — 2000. - Vol. 78, № 4. - P. 413-426.
7. Kennedy SH, Emsley R. Eur Neuropsychopharmacol. 2006;16:93-100.
8. Simon G.E. Long-term prognosis of depression in primary care // Bull. WHO. - — 2000. - Vol. 78, № 4. - P. 439-445.
9. *Post R.M. et al.* Modeling of affective illness // Depression as a lifetime disorder. - Lundbeck, 1994. - — P. 29–51.
10. Izmailova N.T. Depressive disorders in general medical practice and some aspects of their treatment // Med. - – 2002. - №6. - – C. 86 -88
11. Nuller Y.L., Mikhalenko I.N. Affective psychoses. - L.: Medicine, 1988. - — 264 c.
12. Sergeev I.I., Shmilovich A.A., Borodina L.G. Manifestation conditions, clinical and dynamic Phenomenology of phobic disorders // Anxiety and obsessions. - M.: RANS NTSPZ, 1998. - — C. 78–96.
13. Smulevich A.B. Depression in General Medicine. - — M., 2001. - — 252 c.
14. Oganov R.G., Olbinskaya L.I., Smulevich A.B., Vein A.M., Drobizhev M.Y., Shalnova S.A., Pogosova S.A., Shurov D.V. Depression and depressive spectrum disorders in general medical practice. KOMPAS program results // Cardiology. - 2004, № 1. - C.48-54.
15. Negai N.A. Raspopova N.I. Circadian rhythm disorders in the etiopathogenesis of depression and innovative approaches to its effective therapy. - Almaty, 2012- 44 p.
16. Smulevich A.B., Dubnitskaya E. B. Affective diseases of a non-psychotic level - cyclothymia, dysthymia: A manual on psychiatry / Edited by A.S. Liganov. M., 1999. T. 1. C. 608-636.

17. McClung CA. Pharmacol Ther. 2007;114:222-232.
18. Racagni G, Riva MA, Popoli M. Int Clin Psychopharmacol. 2007;22(suppl 2):S9-S14.
19. Nutt D, Wilson S, Paterson L. Dialogues Clin Neurosci. 2008;10:329-336. 20.Mikhaylov B.V. The problem of depression in general somatic practice //.
International Medical Journal. - — M., 2003. - — T. 9, № 3. - — C. 22–27.
21. Andruškevičius S.I. Circadian changes of vegetative activity parameters in depression. // Social and Clinical Psychiatry. 2005; 3: 11-5.
22. Sinton Ch., McCarley V. Neurophysiology and neuropsychiatry of sleep. Neuropsychiatry (Eds. R.B. Schiffer, S.M. Rao, P.S. Fcgel). Philadelphia; Lippincott Williams and Wilkins, 2003: 235-394.
23. Peeters F, Berkhof J, Delespaul P, Rottenberg J, Nicolson NA. Emotion. 2006;6:383-391.
24. Van Someren EJ, Riemersma-Van Der Lek RF. Seep Med Rev. 2007;11:465- 484.
25. Iznak A.F. Modern ideas about neurophysiological bases of depressive disorders. Depression and comorbid disorders / Ed. by A.B.Smulevich. M., 1997. C. 166-179.
26. Kasper S, Hajak G, Wulff K, et al. J Clin Psychiatry. 2010;71:109-120

27. Tiganov A.S. General Psychopathology. Course of lectures. - Moscow: Medical information agency, 2008. - – 197 c.
28. Smulevich A.B. Psychosomatic disorders // Sots. klin. psikhiatr. 1997. № 1.C. 5-18.
29. Popov Y.V., Vid V.D. Clinical psychiatry. SPb, 2004. C. 421.
30. Mikhaylov B.V. The problem of depression in general medical practice //.
International Medical Journal. - — M., 2003. - — T. 9, № 3. - — C. 22–27.
31. Dmitrieva T.B. Polozhyi B.S. History, subject, tasks and methods of social psychiatry Manual on social psychiatry/ Ed. by T.3. Dmitrieva,:. - Moscow: Medicine, 2001. 10-36 p.
32. Tiganov A. S. Affective disorders and syndrome formation // Journal of Neurol. and Psychiatr. 1999. № 1. C. 8-10.
33. Ponizovsky A.M. Masked Depression // The Nurse and Midwife. - – M., 1988. - – №12. C. 36-40
34. ICD-10. Classification of Mental and Behavioral Disorders. Clinical descriptions and guidelines for diagnosis / Translated into Russian and edited by Y.L. Nuller, S.Y. Cirkin. -SPb: Adis, 1994.
35. DSM IV. American Psychiatric Association: Diagnostic and Statistical Manual of Mental Disorders (4 edition). -Washington, DC: APA, 1994
36. Fava M. Depression, somatic symptoms, and antidepressant therapy

(extended abstract). J Clin Psychiatry 2002; 63(4): 305-7.

37. Gerber PD, Barrett JE, Barrett JA et al. The relationship of presenting physical complaints to depressive symptoms in primary care patients. J Gen Intern Med 1992; 7: 170-3.

38. Khlebnikova L.Y. Clinical characteristics of atypical (masked) depressive disorders in patients in general medical practice.

39. Romasenko L.V., Artyukhova M.G., Abramova I.V., Shanayeva I.A. Sleep disorders of different genesis in patients with cardiovascular diseases: Methodological Recommendations. - - M., 2011. - - 22c.

40. Murray G. J Affect Disord. 2007;102:47-53.

41. Dmitrieva T.B., Polozhyi B.S. Social and clinical problems of suicidology in the system of measures to reduce premature mortality and increase the life expectancy of the population. // Bulletin of the Russian Academy of Medical Sciences. - - M., 2006. - №8. - - C. 18-22.

42. Wasserman D. Affective disorders and suicide. Vain death: Causes and prevention of suicide. - - M., 2005. - C. 54-65.

43. Kononchuk N.V. On suicide attempts in depression. // Journal of Neuropathology and Psychiatry. S.S. Korsakov. - 1990. - T. 90, №4. - C. 76-80.

44. Parshin A.N. Suicide risk and clinical diagnosis. // XIV Congress of Psychiatrists of Russia. November 15-18, 2005. (Materials of the congress). - - M., 2005.
- C.445-446.

45. Krasnov V.N. Disorders of the Affective Spectrum. - - M., 2011. - - 431c.

46. Schneider K. Clinical psychopathology. 3 task. Stutgart; G. Thieme Verlag, 1950.

47. Podkorytov V. S., Chaika Yu. Depression and resistance// Journal of Psychiatry and Medical Psychology- 2002. —№ 1.- C. 118-124

48. Altynbekov S.A., Raspopova N.I., Dulyakin E.B. Depressive disorders in general medical practice patients and new possibilities for their effective therapy. Guidelines. - Almaty, 2010. - - 36c.

49. Izmailova N.T., Ilesheva R.G., Kudyarova G.M. Peculiarities of the age aspect of depressive disorders. // Actual questions of psychiatry, narcology and psychology: Collection of scientific works. Almaty, 2000. - - C. 69-72.

50. Smulevich A. B. Clinic and systematics of depression in somatic patients // Sovr. psychiatry. 1998. № 2. C. 4-9.

51. Smulevich A.B. Depression in somatic and mental diseases. - MOSCOW: MIA, 2007. - - C. 72–104.

52. Yanakaeva T.A." Sokolova E.D." Yakhno N.N. Affective cognitive disorders in discirculatory encephalopathy, Alzheimer's disease and Parkinson's disease. Alzheimer's disease and aging: from neurobiology to therapy. M., 1999. C. 156-157.

53. Jenkius R. Depression and anxiety: an overview of preventive strategies // The prevention of depression and anxiety / Eds. R. Jenkius et al. - London: HM Stationary Office, 1992. - — P. 145–157.

54. Averbukh E.S. Depressive states. - — Л., 1962. - — 193 с.

55. Post R.M. et al. Modeling of affective illness // Depression as a lifetime disorder. - Lundbeck, 1994. - — P. 29–51.

56. Lapitsny M.A., Vaulin S. V. Analysis of suicidal behavior, gerontological aspect. Gerontopsychiatry at the turn of the XXI century. M., 1997. C. 38-39.

57. Posvyanskaya A.D. Suicide attempts in patients with depressive disorders. // The Second National Congress of Social Psychiatry "Social Transformations and Mental Health" (Scientific materials). - – M., 2006. - – C.130-131.

58. Petrova N. N., Vanchakova N. P. Factorial value of symptoms included in the diagnostic field of somatized depression: Organizational, clinical and psychological aspects of psychosomatic medicine. SPb., 1996. C. 15-17.

59. Romasenko L.V., Abramova I.V., Artyukhova M.G., Parkhomenko I.M., Diagnosis and therapy of mental disorders in patients in general medical practice. Manual for Doctors. -M., 2006, 31 p.

60. Popov Y.V., Vid V.D. Clinical psychiatry. - SPb., 2002. - — 421 c.

61. Bardenstein L. M. Clinic, dynamics and therapy of dysthymia //. A. Alexandrovsky, L.M. Bardenstein, A.S. Avedisova Psychopharmacotherapy of borderline mental disorders. M., 2000. C. 136-162.

62. Mosolov S.N. Biological mechanisms of recurrent depression and action of antidepressants: new data. Pharmacotherapy of depression. Moscow 2011 pp. 1- 11

63. Snezhnevsky A.V. Clinical psychopathology // Guidance on psychiatry. - — M., 1983. - VOL.1. P. 16-97.

64. Obukhov S.G. Psychiatry, edited by Prof. Y.A. Alexandrovsky - Moscow 2007

65. Selje G. Stress without Distress: Translated from English - M.: Progress, 1979. - — 124 c.

66. BNF 76 Sept 2018-March 2019 Tetracycline antidepressants - P.367.

67. J. Eric Vurphy, K.M. Bridgman. A Comparetive Clinical Trial of Mianserin (Norval) and Amitriptilyne in the Treatment cf Depression in General Practise, J, Inf. Med. Res (1978) 6, 199;

68. Leinonen Esa, Hannu Koponen, Ulla Lepola: Serum mianserin and aging. Neuro-Psychopharmocol. & Biol. Psychiat. 1994, 18(5): 833-845.

69. Forrori M., Lavergno F. et alt., Benefits of mianserin augmentaticn of fluoxetine in patients with major depression non-responders to fluoxetine alone. Acta. Psychiatr. Scand. 2001: 105: 66-72.

70. Murphy J.E. Mianserin in the treatment of depressive illness and anxiety

status in general practice. Br. J. Clin. Pharmac. (1978), 5, 81S-85S;

71. Brogden R.N., Heel R.C., et alt. Mianserin: A Review of the Pharmacological Properties and Therapeutic Efficacy in Depressive Illness. Drags 16: 273-301 (1978).

72. Riemann D. et al. European guideline for the diagnosis and treatment of insomnia. J. Sleep Res. (2017) 26: 680-684.

73. Kelder Jan, Fanke et. alt.: A Comparison of the Phisicochemical and Biological Properties of Mirtazapine and Mianserin. J. Pharm. Pharmacol. 1997. 49; 403-411.

74. Leinonen Esa, Hannu Koponen, Ulla Lepola:Serum mianserin and aging. Neuro-Psychopharmocol. & Biol. Psychiat. 1994, 18(5): 833-845.

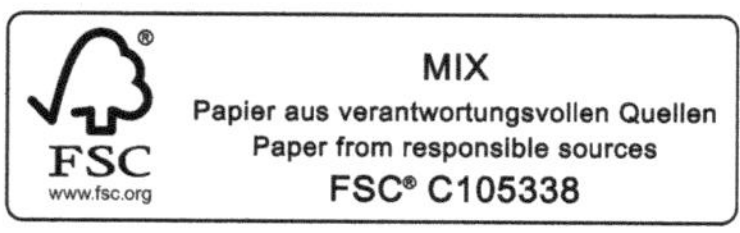

Printed by Books on Demand GmbH, Norderstedt / Germany